Social Work and Social Care

lc|o(

17-5.

Vork and Social Care has been revised and updated to take
count the profound changes that have occurred in social
ver the past two years, in particular the extensive legislative
s to children's and community care services. A new chapter
es the relevance of social exclusion for social work and con-
to affirm the importance of equal opportunities and
scriminatory practice within social work.

oc l Work and Social Care

outlines the importance of social policy for social work
'escribes the powerful ideological forces that underpin current
ractice
considers the future of social work and social care within
a'tered social and political contexts
covers all main areas of social work
includes a glossary and useful website addresses.

This book is essential reading for students approaching the study of
social work, social care and social policy and includes the most
current research available.

Lester Parrott is Senior Lecturer in Social Work at North East
Wales Institute.

The Gildredge Social Policy Series provides introductory textbooks to key areas of policy for the growing number of students of social policy at A level, A/S level, on GNVQ courses, in their first year at university or following a professional diploma course. Written by experienced teachers, the books are short, tightly structured texts designed to be aids to learning.

Series editor: **Pete Alcock**, Professor of Social Policy and Administration, University of Birmingham.

Also in this series:

Education Policy   Paul Trowler
Crime and Social Policy   Mike Stephens
Family Policy   Fran Wasoff and Ian Dey
Health Policy   Ann Wall and Barry Owen
Housing Policy   Jean Conway
The Environment and Social Policy   Michael Cahill

Social Work and Social Care

Second edition

Lester Parrott

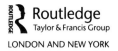

Routledge
Taylor & Francis Group

LONDON AND NEW YORK

First published 1999
by Gildredge

This edition published 2002 by Routledge
2 Park Square, Milton Park, Abingdon, Oxon, OX14 4 RN

Simultaneously published in the USA and Canada
by Routledge
270 Madison Ave, New York, NY 10016

Transferred to Digital Printing 2006

Routledge is an imprint of the Taylor & Francis Group

© 2002 Lester Parrott

Typeset in Times by M Rules
Printed and bound in Great Britain by TJI Digital, Padstow, Cornwall

British Library Cataloguing in Publication Data
A catalogue record for this book is available from the British Library

Library of Congress Cataloging in Publication Data
Parrot, Lester.
    Social work and social care / Lester Parrott. – 2nd ed.
        p. cm. – (The Gildredge social policy series)
    Includes bibliographical references and index.
    1. Social service – Great Britain. 2. Public welfare – Great
Britain. 3. Social service – Government policy – Great Britain. 4.
Great Britain – Social policy. I. Title. II. Series.

HV245 .P28 2002
361.3′2′0941 – dc21   2001052005

ISBN 0–415–23970–2

Contents

Illustrations

Figures

Tables

Foreword

Freddie King, a fine blues singer and guitar wizard, once wrote a song which sums up the problem of relying on the current limited welfare of the state. He wrote, 'What do you do when the welfare walks out on you?' In this country this often means making a trip to the local social services department to try and get some help from a Welfare State that has indeed given up on you. In this context, social work has always been a particularly difficult job. The inherent difficulty of trying to support the poorest, most oppressed sections of this society with few resources, while at the same time having immense legal power to intervene in people's lives, is not merely difficult but impossible at times.

When I first became a social worker in the mid-1970s, the personal social services were just moving out of the post-Seebohm reorganization. Resources were available, and case loads, though high, were mostly tolerable compared to the present. There was the opportunity to become professionally trained and people like me (employed in residential social work at the time) were being seconded on full pay to become professionally qualified. By the time I left the social services in the mid-1990s there was little money, and the constant reduction in local authority resources to meet the increased needs of users led, so it appeared, to wave upon wave of reorganizations as local authorities struggled to manage their dwindling resources. People like me were no longer being seconded and were lucky that they did not have to pay their own tuition fees.

What has happened in this period is part of the story that this book tells, and it is therefore a product of the social, political and economic history which we have all lived through, at best tried to shape, at worst endured.

This book is not exhaustive in that it does not cover all the areas of social work and social care. It is unashamedly a derivative book in that it draws on, in my opinion, some of the key texts in social policy and social work that I and the students I have taught over the years have found most helpful. For the most part, it does not attempt to break any new ground but draws on those texts to develop ideas that remain central to an understanding of social work and social care. There is little mention of juvenile justice or probation, there are no specific chapters on particular user groups in respect of mental health, learning disability or physical disability. This book covers the context in which social work and social care operate socially, politically and economically, drawing on a range of insights from different disciplines.

Foreword to the new edition

Since writing the first edition of this book there have been many changes to the way that the Personal Social Services (PSS) is organized and delivered. New initiatives and policies have come thick and fast and it becomes difficult to keep up with the pace of legislative change and renewal. The changes that have been made to the new edition therefore hopefully capture the transformation that New Labour has wrought within the PSS. I have in the main added to existing chapters where relevant rather than completely change them altogether. I have also updated references where appropriate so that readers will be able to access more contemporary information than was available to me in the first edition. In addition, the glossary has been expanded to cover New Labour's conceptualization of the PSS. Some figures and tables have been updated while others have been removed altogether where they have proved redundant.

Over the past few years the importance of the internet has grown and there have been impressive developments in teaching and learning on the worldwide web which I have also accounted for with an extended list of websites. Readers of the first edition will notice that Chapter 3 has been significantly changed to reflect the importance of social exclusion for social workers who wish to understand the concept and the government's agenda.

Chapter 1, 'Social policy, social work and social care' discusses the importance of social policy analysis for social workers, and argues that social work owes its very existence to the enactment of social policy.

Chapter 2, 'Ideology and the rise of social work' engages with these arguments and examines the ideological nature of social work, from its history from the Poor Law and the struggles to reform it, to the ideological legacy of the New Right.

Chapter 3, 'Anti-discriminatory practice and social exclusion' examines the nature and importance of social exclusion, recognizing the links between ADP and the analysis of social division within social policy. It discusses the importance of social exclusion for New Labour and the role of social work within it.

Chapter 4, 'Residential care: the last resort?' discusses the damaging consequences of viewing residential care as a residual service when all else fails in social work. It looks at current developments in relation to long-term care for older people and the recent legislation in relation to young people leaving care.

Chapter 5, 'Community care' discusses the importance of community care as the policy response to the variety of service users' needs. It stresses the continuity of policy between the Conservatives and New Labour but emphasizes the importance placed by New Labour upon the regulation and control of community care services through the use of managerial approaches to social work.

Chapter 6, 'Policy dilemmas in child and family support' analyses the continuing contradiction inherent in providing support for children and families within an environment which is increasingly rationalizing social work services around the protection of children. It considers the arguments regarding the refocusing of children's services towards a wider assessment of need through the National Assessment Framework and *Quality Protects* (1998).

Chapter 7, 'Citizenship and empowerment' addresses one of the key concerns in modern social work – that of empowering users. It explores the link between ideas of citizenship and that of empowerment. It investigates the problems of community care in this regard, calling on empirical studies which have shown the slow response of local authorities in developing empowering practice.

Chapter 8, 'Social work in altered circumstances' analyses the economic and social context that has changed social work and the Welfare State, and considers New Labour's response in this regard both in general towards the issue of welfare and in particular towards the PSS.

Lester Parrott

Acknowledgements

In writing this new edition there are many people to thank for their support and advice. First in line must be my family. Bernadette shouldered an uneven share of the domestic responsibilities while holding down paid employment. She gave me the encouragement to keep writing while the sun shone and the great outdoors beckoned. Thanks also to Zoe, Frances and Joseph who have shown great understanding and incredible patience when being told for the hundredth time that I couldn't play football with them. Thanks also to Pete Alcock who gave me the chance to write this book originally and offered much sound advice. To all at North East Wales Institute (lecturers and students), who supported me with the time I needed and helpful guidance, particularly the students who bought the first book, here's hoping you buy this one. Finally, thanks to all at Routledge, particularly Edwina Welham who has provided much e-mail support and the opportunity for writing the new edition. Any errors and failure to acknowledge sources of information are of course mine and I apologize in advance for any mistakes made in this regard.

Chapter 1

Social policy, social work and social care

OUTLINE
This chapter will:

● discuss the development of social policy, its definition and its relationship with social work
● examine the relationship between social work and the state
● outline the main areas of social work
● describe the value dilemmas involved in social work practice.

From social administration to social policy

Social policy has been closely linked with social work since the first social work students were trained at the London School of Economics at the beginning of the twentieth century. Social policy was presented as an administrative and organizational discipline concerned with giving students the knowledge to manage welfare efficiently, teaching students how to be social administrators so that they could better operate the emerging welfare services. Debate about how appropriate the current welfare system was came second to the task of improving existing welfare provision, the principles of which were taken for granted. To talk of social policy at this stage would be misleading; the subject area was social administration.

Throughout the early part of the twentieth century, research into welfare focused on how poverty was implicated in a range of social problems. Researchers measured need in order to provide the technical information upon which policy-makers could act. Questions about how need should be defined or responded to were not the stuff of social administration. This approach reached its zenith during and after the Second World War when governments commissioned social research to plan the war effort and subsequently construct the post-war Welfare State.

From 1945 to the early 1970s, social administration operated within a social and political consensus that the state should take considerable responsibility for the welfare of its citizens. It developed for the most part within narrow policy parameters, which accepted rather than questioned the nature of this compromise and the role that welfare played within it. This compromise has often been referred to as the 'post-war consensus' or 'settlement'. The ruling sections of the major political parties, the civil service, representatives of industry and the trade unions generally agreed that the continued expansion of the Welfare State was in all their interests. The dominant issue for the discipline of social administration was how to develop the Welfare State by refining government policy within this broad agreement.

By the early 1970s, the consensus around the Welfare State and the role of social administration within it began to fragment. Critics from a variety of ideological positions began to doubt the basic assumptions upon which the Welfare State and social administration were based. Marxist, New Right and feminist writers, for example, began to unpick the policies and major assumptions upon which the post-war settlement had nourished the expansion of the state into welfare. As a result, a more critical and sociological conception of the study of welfare developed – social policy widened the question of welfare beyond the confining limits of social administration.

What is social policy?

Social policy studies not only the organization and delivery of state welfare services, but also how well-being can be promoted within society generally. Well-being may be achieved through the satisfaction of individuals' socially defined needs. Although adequacy of food, shelter and clothing may seem to be an unambiguous measure of need, these needs are expressed differently by people from different cultures and societies. If we take into account people's psychological and emotional development, the issue becomes more complex and presents social policy with new challenges. If, for example, parents cannot leave their children to play safely in the street for fear of a car accident or abduction, their sense of well-being is affected. These questions require us to be clear at what level and to what extent the Welfare State can and should satisfy need.

At one level we can take a more inclusive view and include differences of culture, taste and the so-called higher emotional and psychological needs; or we can use a restrictive approach, which keeps the satisfaction of needs at a basic level, usually focusing on food, shelter and clothing. These questions move beyond the academic when we consider how far the state should satisfy the needs of specific individuals. How much, for example, should the state allocate in social security benefits to meet the needs of those unable to maintain themselves? Should the present basic level of income support be increased to meet the wider social and psychological needs of claimants? How much recognition of different needs between claimants should there be? Should the extra costs incurred in being a single parent/carer or a person with a physical disability be taken into account? By limiting benefit payment for these extra costs, those affected face significant barriers to participate fully in society.

Social policy does not content itself only with academic considerations; it also aims to improve social conditions. To do so it has to consider appropriate social action; inevitably value judgements have to be made in choosing between one course of action over another. This presents a dilemma for social policy between analysis and practice; as Erskine (1997, p. 14) suggests, 'analysis requires scepticism while practice requires conviction'.

Issues for social policy

In understanding the concept of well-being, social policy uses the methods of a number of social science disciplines to engage with social problems in a rigorous and scientific way. Deciding what action to take means choosing between alternatives and taking sides. This raises dilemmas 'which social science cannot resolve' (Erskine 1997, p. 7). Social science can inform and guide us by clarifying the reasons for choice, but it cannot make the choice for us.

Social policy has to consider:

● well-being – not just as a product of government action, but as a result of social factors.

It is impossible to assess the contribution of people caring for others if our focus is purely on the caring services provided by the state. The majority of care in society is delivered informally, mostly by women, and makes an enormous contribution to the overall level of well-being in society.

Social policy therefore considers:

● who provides welfare, which groups benefit from it, and, particularly, how access is denied to some groups.

The informal care provided by women comes at a cost of forgone careers, time, emotional effort and so on. This unrecognized labour benefits government and saves the Welfare State considerable expense.

● the impact of welfare on the overall distribution of power and wealth in society.

Providing unpaid and unrecognized care restricts women to the private sphere of the family, enabling men to achieve recognition and power in the public sphere of work. This increases women's dependence upon men, and effectively limits their opportunity to acquire income and wealth independently.

Social difference

In recent years, social policy has begun to study the concept of social difference, i.e. how the social location of the providers and users of services affects their experience of welfare. It looks at those groups who have been marginalized by society, and studies their everyday experience of welfare. It attempts to link their personal and often private experiences with the public face of social policy. Recently, marginalized groups, such as people with disabilities, single parents and people from ethnic minorities, have demanded that their voice be heard in the policy-making process. As a result, their demands are making some impact on the policy-making process and the delivery of welfare. For many writers, the concept of social difference has become a key theme in the analysis of social policy. Chapter 3 looks more closely at these issues.

Social work and social policy

Social work and social policy share a commitment to social change. Social work addresses issues of:

- individual rights to welfare
- the rights of the individual and the expectations of society
- challenging inequality and oppression experienced by users
- justice in social policy.

Both social work and social policy have experienced radical change. Social policy has broadened its approach to take into account the diversity of people's experiences and the essentially contested nature of the Welfare State. Social work, in developing anti-discriminatory approaches, seeks to put this theoretical knowledge of difference into practice. This demands an approach that understands people's personal problems within a broader social context and uses this knowledge to effect change both for individuals and their social environment. Figure 1.1 shows the interface between social work and social policy.

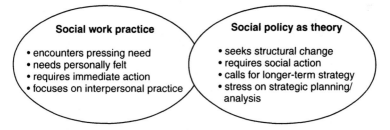

Social work practice
- encounters pressing need
- needs personally felt
- requires immediate action
- focuses on interpersonal practice

Social policy as theory
- seeks structural change
- requires social action
- calls for longer-term strategy
- stress on strategic planning/ analysis

Figure 1.1 Social work and social policy

For students approaching social work, social policy explains both the social circumstances of the users of social work services, and the social work organizations themselves. Social policy can therefore explain how social work as a service is:

- produced – through a mixed economy of care
- consumed – with differences in how social work and social care services are experienced and accessed by users
- distributed – with unequal distribution of services between different classes, age groupings or ethnic groups.

Case study

Mr Amarnath has been on Income Support for three years. Recently, his cooker finally broke down, and he cannot afford to buy another one without help from the Social Fund. He approaches his local social services department for advice as to how he should apply.

Commentary
A social worker cannot effectively approach the social security system on behalf of a user without a working knowledge of its organization. An uninformed approach to the Social Fund could result in Mr Amarnath being unsuccessful in his application. Mr Amarnath's social worker will have learned from the research that has investigated how the social security system operates to provide clients with, or prevent them from receiving, an adequate income (Kempson 1996). Of particular relevance are the studies on the social security system's failure to recognize and meet the needs of black people (Law 1996, Chapter 2). Further, knowledge of the social security system will be of little use unless social workers can place its provision within the wider social context of support (or lack of it) from other agencies.

This case study shows the importance of social policy for social work in three key areas:

1 knowledge of how users experience the social context
2 knowledge that enables social workers to intervene effectively on behalf of users
3 knowledge of the context in which social work operates, in terms of the law, policy, procedures and organizations involved.

Social policy and social work education

Since 1989, increasing emphasis on the development of the basic roles and tasks of social workers has narrowed the definition of what should be included in the social work training curriculum. More recently, a further attempt to limit the field of social work education along narrow occupational lines has focused more attention on the practical skills and knowledge required (for example, knowledge of the law in social work). The power of the previous Conservative government over the professional bodies in social work has been crucial in forcing the pace of change. Conservative ministers were increasingly concerned that social work educators and social workers were focusing on anti-discriminatory practice rather than on delivering what the government considered to be a social work service free of what they considered to be political and ideological bias. Or as Jones (1996) has argued, the Conservatives desired a social work service that did not engage critically with the increasing social inequality and injustice which had been a marked feature of the Conservative Party's approach to the PSS (see Chapter 3).

The recently defined standards for qualifications in social work require social work educators to teach a narrow range of skills and knowledge. This has led to social work courses cutting back on the teaching of such subjects as social policy and sociology, in favour of subjects considered to be more occupationally relevant. While demanding more of social work education, the Conservative government maintained the period of training at two years rather than three. The current government has now confirmed a three-year programme for social work education which will mean social work will become a graduate profession similar to that of nursing. Although the content of social work education is likely to reflect a continuing emphasis upon skills development which is important to providing competent social workers, understanding the wider social context in which social work operates must not be seen as a luxury. Understanding the social context in which social workers work with users is crucial. It contributes to the repertoire of values, skills and knowledge that social workers must use in an imaginative and critically informed way. It also militates against the uninformed 'common-sense' approach to social work that is often argued for by the media and some politicians, particularly around issues of race (Alibhai-Brown 1993). Social policy, as part of a critical endeavour, enables social workers to move beyond the common-sense reality of the proponents of the new, practical social work. Theoretically informed and critical practice is better placed to understand the complexity of individuals' social relations, and the significance this has for themselves and for society.

The regulation of the social work profession

To control the content of social work training is a powerful instrument in determining the kind of social work professional society wants, as what students learn on their courses will, it is assumed, determine the kinds of skills, values and knowledge they will take with them as qualified professionals. It is therefore impossible to discuss the regulation of the social work profession as distinct from that of social work education itself. The Care Standards Act 2000 represents a significant step in defining the standards that social work professionals must acquire and enforces those standards through the compulsory registration of social workers and regulation of the content of their training. Thus the Care Council will become the regulating body which will:

- enforce codes of conduct and practice standards applying to all social care staff in whatever sector they work
- codes of practice will be enforced with employers in whatever sector they employ care staff
- register individuals, set the entry requirements for registration and exclude or suspend those for misconduct and bad practice.

Crucial to this enterprise for the government is that the membership of the Council will be constituted by a majority of lay members representing not only service users but employers as well. This is in contrast to many other professional bodies where the professional representation dominates; for example, doctors' and nurses' bodies within the medical profession. While the involvement of service users is welcome it will require the lay members to have a real working knowledge of the issues involved in regulating professional bodies particularly in relation to education and training. This may be a welcome move forward given the problems of professionals regulating themselves (for example, the Shipman case in relation to the medical profession), yet social work professionals have never wielded as much power as the more entrenched professions such as doctors and lawyers. However, to give almost total control to lay members and employers in the process may also lose valuable professional input into the process. This is likely to bring its own problems, as Davies (2000) argues, where social work professionals could be left in a kind of limbo with little power to question and challenge the method of regulation.

Social work and the state

Government expenditure on the personal social services (PSS) is a small proportion of the Welfare State budget, as shown in Table 1.1.

Table 1.1 UK state spending on Welfare State services 1997–1998

	Spending to nearest £billion
Social security	131
Housing	6
PSS	10
Health	44
Education	36
Total	227

Source: Central Statistical Office 2000

Most people will have little or no contact with the PSS, compared with the education and health services. According to Baldock (1997), at any one time a local social services department will be working with:

- one third of those over 85 years old
- less than 4 per cent of children in families living on benefit
- less than 2 per cent of children with physical disabilities
- less than 10 per cent of those with a mental illness and supported in the community.

There is therefore a considerable social distance between social work and the majority of the population. Most people can describe with reasonable accuracy the work of a doctor, nurse or teacher, yet have difficulty describing what a social worker does. This is confirmed by the Social Service Inspectorate/Audit Commission (1998) which show that even in the best performing local authorities only one-third of people have information about social services before they use them.

Social work and social care as a professional activity are indeed hard to define. The area is diverse, changeable and politically controversial. Social work is scattered across different sites, working with different sorts of people. As Parton (1996a) argues, the problem of description is one of social work's defining characteristics, for it is 'in an essentially contested and ambiguous position'. It is contested, for social work has always been the subject of argument and debate concerning its purpose in society; it is ambiguous, for it operates between 'individual initiative and the all encompassing state' (Parton 1996a, p. 6).

As noted above, social workers have to balance the rights of individual service users with their statutory responsibilities coupled with the requirement to challenge unjust policies as they affect users. Any definition of social work and social care has to recognize that its power to operate is circumscribed by law. Parliament outlines how social workers should respond to certain groups of individuals. Legislation can, for example, place a duty upon social services departments to act to prevent child abuse, while giving them considerable discretion with regard to family support. In assessing whether children are at risk, the law requires social workers to use their professional judgement in deciding whether to intervene in a situation. Social workers have been heavily criticized, particularly by the media and some politicians, for intervening either too quickly or not quickly enough (see Chapter 6).

In operating on behalf of the state, workers in the PSS are involved in a balancing act; they are required to represent the state to users of services with whom they work, while advocating on behalf of individuals back to the state. In the UK (unlike other countries, such as Germany), social workers are required to carry out statutory and protective roles, while at the same time promoting social justice. In Germany this contradiction is resolved by employing both social workers (with a protective role) and social pedagogues (with an enabling community role). Both functions are legitimated by the state with qualification in one specialism not preventing entry to the other, while in the UK social workers and community workers are trained separately (Jeffries and Muller 1997).

A mixed economy of welfare

The personal social services include:

- social work – needs assessment, preventive and protective work with adults and children
- provision of group care – residential and day care
- community care services – provision of domiciliary and social support
- youth offending – work within multidisciplinary teams to prevent youth crime.

These activities reflect the organizational context within which state-funded social work and social care is carried out. They make up the range of professional services provided by the state. At the same time, these services are increasingly provided by the private and voluntary (independent) sectors, supplemented by an informal sector (family/neighbour care).

Social work has always struggled for legitimacy within the Welfare State. Following the Second World War, universal services such as health and education were established as core provisions available to all. Social work, on the other hand, was conceived as a final safety net, on which people would rely when all else had failed. It was not until 1968 that the Seebohm Report conceived the PSS as something more than this. Seebohm proposed the creation of a fifth social service which would be available to all citizens on a universal basis. This commitment, as Chapter 2 will show, was short-lived, and social work continues to struggle with its residual role.

Since the late 1970s, the main political parties have increasingly seen state provision of PSS as one arm of a mixed economy of welfare, including the independent and informal sectors. The National Health Service and Community Care Act 1990 (NHSCCA 1990) confirmed this trend by requiring local authorities to transfer the bulk of existing service provision to the private and voluntary sectors. The Local Government Act 1999 reinforces this trend by requiring local authorities to deliver PSS through a mixed economy of care to achieve value for money and quality outcomes, described as Best Value.

The role of the local authority social services department has therefore changed; it now co-ordinates a diversity of provision through a number of providers. Because this has profoundly affected the way social workers carry out their tasks, managerial responses are assuming increasing importance. Social workers are predominantly co-ordinators of packages of care, managing the process of service provision rather than working directly with users. The following case study is an example of how independent and informal care may combine with state provision.

Case study

Mrs Davies is 85 years old and lives on her own in a warden-controlled flat. She attends a local luncheon club run by Age Concern in her local church hall twice a week. To help her around the home she pays for a private home help service to clean and shop for her, some four hours a week. Any other support is provided by her daughter who visits twice a week. Every three months she goes into a local authority residential home for a fortnight's respite care where her progress is assessed, and any future needs are addressed with her care manager.

Who is providing care for Mrs Davies?

- state sector – respite care, care management and assessment of need, warden-controlled housing
- voluntary sector – Age Concern
- private sector – home help service
- informal sector – her daughter's visits.

Social work as an occupation

Social work is divided into four main occupational groupings:

1 field social work
2 residential and day care work
3 social care work
4 welfare rights and community development.

These divisions differ not only in their functions, but also in the resources and political support they attract; they have unequal professional status, pay and conditions of service. This has been particularly marked in local authority social work, and to some extent in the voluntary sector. Field social workers are the most privileged, in occupational terms, compared to those in the residential and social care sectors. These divisions have become more marked as the role of the private sector has increased in residential and domiciliary care, further undercutting pay and working conditions within local authorities.

Social work, social care, residential care and welfare rights/ community work deliver services in the following settings:

- *Day centres.* Day centres are attended on a daily basis by people with different social, social education and training needs (which are not usually grouped together). Older people, for example, who are unable to move out of their own homes, join together for social activities; people with learning disabilities attend a social education and training programme on basic living and social skills to help them live independently in the community.
- *Residential care.* People may live in residential care over the long term (for example, older people, children in care), or for a short period to give themselves and/or their carers a break.
- *Social services offices.* These cover a given geographical area and are usually divided between children's services and adult services. Social work is the provision of direct services, such as case management and assessing people's need for services. A social worker might arrange ongoing social support, involving advice and guidance around a particular life crisis, such as

bereavement. Such help may involve advocacy on behalf of a person with another agency upon whose services they rely, for example, making a claim for social security benefits. Social care, on the other hand, is the provision of services to people in their homes. This is provided by domiciliary services to support people unable to manage basic living tasks, for example, shopping or general housework. However, as social workers take on more case-management work, social care is becoming increasingly involved in general social support and basic assessment.

Social workers make up a privileged minority of the labour force within the PSS; Figure 1.2 shows the disparity in levels of qualification for different occupational groups.

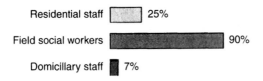

Figure 1.2 Percentage of local authority staff professionally qualified, by occupational grouping

- *Welfare rights and community work.* This may occur in a variety of settings. Welfare rights workers are usually in their own separate units, engaging with the variety of social security problems presented by those users who are overwhelmingly dependent upon state benefits. Increasingly, benefits are being used to enhance the incomes of people in an attempt to compensate them for the growth in charging for welfare services. Community work is less available within the PSS than it was in the 1970s. The early enthusiasm for community development within social work departments has waned as local authorities have sought, in the face of increased demand, to focus provision on their statutory responsibilities.

Value dilemmas and the purpose of social work

Case study

Mrs Phillips is 80 years old. She lives on her own and draws a state pension combined with a disability living allowance. She is having increasing problems living in her own home and requires more domiciliary care. Her social worker visits, but was told by the social work manager that Mrs Phillips has reached the spending limit for domiciliary care and it will now be cheaper to offer residential care. If Mrs Phillips requires more home care, she will have to pay for it herself. The social worker knows that she does not have the money to do this. Mrs Phillips is fiercely independent and does not want to consider any form of residential care. The social worker's conclusion is that she would be able to remain at home if more domiciliary hours were available.

Commentary

This situation highlights the dilemma between upholding a user's right to a particular lifestyle and the requirement to follow particular departmental policies that may limit these rights. A social worker may assess a person for a service to keep them living in their own home and yet find that, because of resource constraints, the services required cannot be met from the existing budget of the social services department. What can social workers and social care workers do in this situation? As employees of the social service department, do they:

- accept the constraints placed upon them?
- have a duty to advocate on behalf of the person they have assessed to have their needs met in full?
- challenge the legislation and legal judgments that prevent them from providing an effective service for users?

These dilemmas are at the core of an activity that attempts to mediate between the needs of an individual and the state's statutory and resource requirements. In this instance, the social worker should do everything possible to enable Mrs Phillips to live with dignity in her own home by, in the first instance, advocating back to the department about the importance of domiciliary provision. Social workers and social care workers are constantly faced with similar situations, which present them with profound ethical dilemmas.

Webb and Wistow (1987) argue that social work contributes to one or more of three basic functions:

● social control
● the promotion of change
● social maintenance.

Social control

Most social workers are paid employees of the state and are expected to perform certain statutory duties on behalf of society. These duties bring them into contact with certain acts which society regards as deviant and may sometimes lead to conflicting imperatives within the worker's role. Although these duties generally have the wider support of society, problems arise as to the best way to carry them out. An example is child protection; there may be general agreement that children should be protected from abuse, but there is no real consensus as to how. An over-emphasis on protecting children (perhaps by taking them into care) may, if it is carried out to the detriment of the general support of the family, create more problems than it prevents. If basic social support is not provided, over-protection may create greater stress for families, resulting in the breakdown of relationships, which in turn can lead to further abuse of children. The best way to protect children in these situations is therefore contested and often confused. Some people demand that social workers should provide more support for families and concentrate on keeping them together. Others see social workers as the dupes of the abusers, failing to provide children with the protection to which they are entitled. Media coverage of two such cases highlights these issues well in relation to Derbyshire and Haringey Social Services where social workers and their managers have been reported as failing in their assessments of abusive carers who subsequently murdered children in their care. Social work has to balance the need to care for individuals and families with the duty, at times, to intervene in order to control particular behaviours and situations. As Webb and Wistow (1987) suggest, this can lead to three possible responses.

Response 1

Should social work be involved in controlling behaviour at all? Should not social workers always respect the free will of individuals with whom they work and enable them to make their own decisions?

This approach has to some extent influenced the debate about empowerment, where a social worker's duty to intervene and make decisions on behalf of individuals is seen as illegitimate and unnecessary (see Chapter 7).

In some areas social workers will use their statutory powers to limit free choice of certain individuals in order to protect the choices of others. Paedophilia is one example where social workers and the police intervene to prevent some adults from exercising their preference for sexual contact with children, in order to keep children free from harm.

Response 2

If it is accepted that social control is necessary in some situations, what forms of control are appropriate for particular situations?

Some discharged patients from mental health hospitals have subsequently been involved in murder and serious physical assaults, and this has led to criticism of the support available to those being rehabilitated into the community. New legislation will involve greater control, such as requiring people to undergo compulsory treatment in the community if they fail to take prescribed medication. Opponents argue that this will infringe the human rights of individuals in the community; existing legislation can be used to enforce treatment in hospital already. The issue is not whether to control, but how.

Response 3

Should social workers exercise social control in a society that is unjustly divided along lines such as class, race and gender? The focus here is not on the social control of individuals, but on the lack of social justice, which excludes marginalized groups from society. For example, when social workers are assessing older people who may need help in their own homes, should they take into account the ability of relatives to care for them, or would this be abdicating the state's responsibility? Does this in turn shift the duty of care on to relatives, and in particular female relatives, so further reinforcing gender divisions? Investigation of the way in which social work supports or challenges the social order inevitably raises questions about the balance of social and economic power in society. It leads us to ask questions about who needs services, why access is denied to certain groups and why some groups are subject to more punitive treatment than others (see Chapter 3).

In highlighting the debate over social control and social work it is important to emphasize that the use of social control is not always a negative aspect of social work. In many areas, such as child abuse work or mental health work, social control may be used positively to defend the rights of individuals who may lack an adequate voice of their own. This means that social workers will exercise power at times to intervene in the personal lives of others, for example, to protect one member of a family against the illegitimate power and force of another. Social control used in this way can be a positive intervention, to promote justice and equality between individuals in areas that are often concealed from the public gaze.

Promotion of social change

Social work promotes change at the individual and social level, but writers on social work disagree as to which of these should be emphasized (see Chapter 3). The development of anti-discriminatory practice (ADP) is a response to this controversy. It provides a perspective for social work that seeks to understand the impact of oppression upon people's lives. In breaking from purely individualistic practices that attempt to alter the individual's personality or particular emotional state, ADP develops a model for understanding the different experiences of individuals from diverse social backgrounds. Issues of gender and race, for example, influence and provide a framework for the way in which people experience their world. It requires social workers to assess their own practice and employing organization to determine how effectively they may be responding to the different needs of service users. Law (1996) shows the gross disparity in resources going towards people from ethnic minorities within the PSS. Anti-discriminatory practice requires social workers to take positive steps to address this inequality by changing their own practice if required and the organizations they work for.

While this approach promises to promote change, it is too narrow if the users of such services are excluded. Including the users of services means working in partnership to change the way services are developed and provided. The aim is to focus on the needs of users, rather than the political agenda of government, or the needs of social service organizations. It should enable service users to have a central role in this process and as such question any approach to ADP that places social work professionals at the epicentre of practice (Wilson and Beresford 2000).

Social maintenance

The importance of social maintenance as a function of social work and social care has grown as services concentrate upon supporting people in their communities. It involves services designed to care for individuals in a way that maintains an acceptable quality of life. These services, which involve social and domestic support and personal care, are often the most popular in the PSS. They maintain people in the community who would otherwise have to move into some form of institutional care, or fall back to an even greater extent on any family they may have. Increasingly the control of this function and the assumption of care has been challenged. The

Disability Movement has called for the greater use of direct payments for social care so that disabled people themselves are given their own budget for the help they need. This enables greater choice as to what kind of care they receive, when and how it is delivered. The notion of social maintenance as care is criticized by disabled people who argue that this creates dependence; they demand control over the assistance they need to enable them to become autonomous citizens (Morris 1997).

The skills involved in social care have not always been recognized by social work professionals, particularly by those who argue that it involves less complex skills and tasks. Social care has been devalued as the junior partner of social work, lacking the same professional complexity. This distinction is false. The provision of effective social care services demands an awareness and understanding of personal relationships and social issues similar to that involved in social work. Twigg (2000) provides an interesting study of social care and bathing, suggesting that washing and bathing are far from straightforward or commonsensical in the significance they have for those experiencing them.

Conclusion

This chapter has described the complex relationship between social policy and social work. Both draw on a range of social science disciplines which provide the possibility of effecting real change for those excluded from society. Social policy, alongside sociology and psychology, provides the underpinning knowledge to enable social work to go beyond the confines of common-sense solutions to social problems. The insights that social policy offers combined with the skills of social work and a commitment to anti-discriminatory practice holds out the possibility for an integrated and effective practice.

Key points

- Social work and social policy share a commitment to social change.
- Social policy, as part of an integrated approach to knowledge, informs effective social work practice.

● Social work mediates between excluded individuals and society.
● Social policy, with its concern for issues of race, class and gender, informs social work's commitment to anti-discriminatory practice.

Guide to further reading

For a succinct introductory text on social policy, Alcock, P. (1996) *Social Policy in Britain*, London: Macmillan, provides a useful beginning. For a discussion of some of the key issues covered in this book, but in greater depth, Parton, N. (ed.) (1996c) *Social Theory, Social Change and Social Work*, London: Routledge, comprises a number of excellent chapters written by leading authorities in social work and social policy. Thompson, N. (1998) *Promoting Equality: Challenging Discrimination and Oppression in the Human Services*, London: Macmillan, provides a deeper understanding of anti-discriminatory practice.

Chapter 2

Ideology and the rise of social work

OUTLINE
This chapter will:

- define ideology and analyse its importance for social work
- investigate the influence of New Right and Fabian ideologies
- describe the history of social work and the influence of Fabian and New Right thinking
- examine the changes to social work in the 1980s.

What is ideology?

Giddens (2001) defines ideology as a system of shared ideas serving to justify the interests of dominant groups in society. Ideologies are important to social policy because they shape the way we understand, for example:

- the nature of social work
- the users of welfare services
- the nature of welfare organizations
- the value and purpose of social work within the Welfare State.

The term ideology has been used in two ways in social policy.

1   *Ideology as a critical concept*
    Ideology is used critically by evaluating an existing set of ideas and values that claim to explain the nature of the social world in which we live. Marxists, for example, suggest that capitalism as an ideology conceals the real nature of exploitation in society. The ruling class exercises its power over society by using false ideas about the nature of the social system we live in to hide the injustice of that system from the rest of the population.

2   *Ideology as a descriptive concept*
    A range of competing ideologies is described without necessar-
    ily giving priority to one system of ideas over any other.
    They are descriptive devices used to analyse competing ideas and
    their relative influence upon social policy.

Social policy usually adopts the second sense, and studies the
impact of ideologies on the making of social policy, although some
writers will be less committed to this view than others. Marxists
analyse all such statements as ideological in themselves; they would
claim that social policy, by not adopting a critical stance, may mask
an ideological viewpoint under the guise of maintaining descriptive
neutrality.

For an ideology to affect society it must:

● have a clear view on human nature – what motivates individuals
   to behave and think the way they do
● describe reality in a reasonably coherent and logical fashion –
   its descriptions of social situations must make 'sense', by telling
   a story that explains current events convincingly; this description is often a critique of the existing social order
● provide a vision of the future – by offering hope of a better
   world
● provide guidance on how to change the current order – by providing a call to action and a blueprint for change.

This chapter analyses New Right and Fabian approaches. These
are not the only ideological perspectives within social work, but
they usefully highlight some of the key debates around the role of
the individual and the state in social work. It is important to recog-
nise that by focusing upon the individual and the state, these
ideologies say nothing about the differences between individuals,
for example, in terms of race and gender. Chapter 3 investigates
anti-discriminatory approaches that take such differences into
account. Further, neither the New Right nor the Fabian approaches
describe perspectives that may cut across the two extremes of the
individual and the state. Chapter 8 considers the example of the
'Third Way' associated with New Labour as an approach in which
elements of both pro-state and pro-individual ideologies combine;

the 'Third Way' both formulates a role for government in reforming the Welfare State, and at the same time emphasizes responsibility for meeting welfare needs by individuals themselves. Tables 2.1 and 2.2 outline the basic positions of the New Right and Fabianism.

Table 2.1 The New Right

Human nature. Individuals require both freedom to choose and incentives to do well. They must accept the consequences of these choices if unsuccessful.

The state should practise minimum interference; government must encourage free enterprise, be strong in terms of law and order, and conserve existing institutions and morality, e.g. the nuclear family, 'traditional values', such as respect for authority.

The Welfare State must encourage independence and self-help, e.g. private health insurance, voluntary activity; it must control behaviour which challenges traditional values or institutions, e.g. having children outside marriage.

Community is spontaneous; it develops through individual and family attachments in small local neighbourhoods.

Social work. Pragmatic activity must encourage independence by working alongside voluntary and private sectors; ideally, social workers are employed by the private sector, to work with those in greatest need.

Table 2.2 Fabianism

Human nature. People are social, not purely individual beings; society should organize to strengthen solidarity and community cohesion.

The state is more efficient than the market, and should attempt to create equality and social justice by reducing extremes of income and wealth.

The Welfare State is the vehicle to promote altruism, solidarity and community by providing universal social services to all.

Table 2.2 continued

Community. Left to themselves, communities can be destroyed by individualism; community has to be nurtured and developed by the state.

Social work. The state service should provide universal non-stigmatizing social services. It should recognize that some individuals may need specialist help due to their inability to function in a modern society.

The development of social work

The poor law

Social work developed in the UK as a response to the individual and social problems associated with living in an acquisitive capitalist society. This development was not unproblematic or inevitable, but reflected the twin processes of rapid industrialization and urbanization in the nineteenth century. These processes radically changed the social circumstances in which people were employed – increasingly in factories – and where they were housed – in large urban centres that attracted people in search of work. For those considered unfit for the demands placed upon them by the new factory system, and for those periodically unemployed, the consequences were harsh – more so since the old systems of support were considered too costly by the new entrepreneurial classes, who required flexible, cheap labour. Their solution was to develop a system of minimum support that would encourage the able-bodied poor to support themselves.

The Poor Law (Amendment) Act 1834 was such a system. For believers in the new society, the traditional relationships of custom and obligation encouraged dependency and a lack of personal responsibility. A developing industrial society required people to be mobile and to take their own chances in life.

The principle behind the new Poor Law was to reduce eligibility for relief (assistance), by keeping relief below the level that the lowest labourer could earn in work; people would therefore choose to work. This was reinforced by the shame of losing personal freedom, since relief was available only in the workhouse. Less eligibility and indoor relief would provide the perfect mechanism to enhance the working of the market. The spectre of the workhouse would not only deter the lazy and workshy, but would encourage those in work to make their own provision, through forms of private insurance provided by savings banks and friendly societies. Those who were poor through no 'fault' of their own, such as widows or the old, could be granted outdoor relief; the workhouse thus became a place for 'moral failures'.

The new Poor Law created a distinction between the deserving and the undeserving poor that stigmatized the destitute who had to rely on it. The mark of shame that attached to those in the workhouse became the key deterrent for the able-bodied poor, as the poorest labourer often earned less than the meagre support provided by the workhouse. Rigid and petty rules categorizing and controlling the inmates within the workhouse reinforced their feelings of stigma. This affected even 'deserving cases'; as life expectancy increased through the century, greater numbers of older people were forced into the workhouses.

The situation scandalized many supporters of the Poor Law; they saw unfortunate individuals with previous 'sound characters' forced through unemployment to enter the workhouse. Many charitable organizations responded to prevent such people from feeling the shame of indoor relief. However, with the expansion of charitable work came the fear that without proper organization the objectives of these organizations might be diluted by indiscriminate giving, resulting in the feckless and lazy receiving help. This view provided the spur to establish the Charity Organization Society (COS) in 1869, whose sponsors maintained that assistance should be given according to the principles of the Poor Law. The COS wished to organize the various charitable bodies throughout the country to provide help in a systematic and co-ordinated way.

The core of the philosophy of the COS was a belief in the personal advancement of the poor through self-help. It was an attempt to create a discretionary approach to the failures of character which were held to be at the root of poverty. The COS, through systematic examination of people's circumstances and motivation, would ensure that only the deserving would receive help. It would also identify those who applied for help with little intention of self-improvement as candidates for the workhouse. To meet these aims, volunteers were recruited to investigate and act as role models for the poor, by dispensing advice and by force of example. The techniques in this moral surveillance were to form the basis of a general approach in social work, whereby the supplicants for help were interviewed and assessed, and their backgrounds recorded in case notes and files. Casework was not to be entered into by the untutored; it had to be approached scientifically, by the application of rational principles that required a detached approach. The COS developed basic training courses in these investigative techniques, leading to the setting up of a School of Sociology in 1902 to train social workers in the methods and philosophy of the COS.

Many middle-class women, who were denied participation in the public world of the late nineteenth century, found charitable help attractive. While the administration of charity was placed firmly in the hands of men, a growing number of women found an outlet for their aspirations for employment and public service as visitors to the poor. This gender difference between managers and practitioners has proved to be remarkably tenacious in social work to the present day.

Liberalism and Fabianism

While the COS continued to work alongside the Poor Law, a challenge to the explanation of poverty on individual grounds was developed by two competing sections of the middle classes. First, in the early 1860s, the Liberal Party moved away from the individualistic philosophy that had dominated its political thought in the early 1800s. This new liberalism was set out in J.S. Mill's book *Principles of Political Economy*, a radical critique of classical liberal political economy. It led, by the 1880s and 1890s, to new liberal writers becoming closely aligned with socialists in criticizing the extremes of poverty and wealth in Victorian society (Clarke *et al.* 1987). Second, the Fabian Society was founded in 1883 with the aim of propagating collectivist principles in Britain. It challenged the prevailing orthodoxy of the free market by sustained campaigning. The Society wanted to achieve its goal by methodical evolutionary means, through the power of persuasion and gradual adoption of socialist policy in government. Its attitude to the poor was in many respects similar to that of the COS, which, as Morris (1994) argues, viewed the destitute as a danger to the evolution of socialism.

Sidney Webb, one of the key figures within the society, was clear that while capitalist society was inefficient and ethically wrong, the destitute were morally inferior, 'degenerate hordes of a demoralized "residuum" unfit for social life' (Morris 1994, p. 26). These opinions formed the mainstream thought; middle-class Victorians shared a fear of those who were, in their opinion, genetically unfit, i.e. those labelled lunatics and idiots or so-called moral defectives, such as unmarried mothers. The Fabians, like the COS, feared that such people had the potential to threaten the human stock of British society. They argued that if these dangerous classes were not checked, then the intelligence and moral character of the nation would be tarnished.

Unlike the COS, the Fabians regarded the organization and administration of the Poor Law as inefficient and ineffective. For the Fabians, belief in the rational scientific control of society by the state was paramount. They wished to see society governed by an administrative elite who could manage society judiciously for the greater good of all. The COS, on the other hand, wished to reinforce the voluntary principle within the Poor Law system. Between the margins of casework and social administration that the COS and the Fabians promoted as the solution to poverty and moral decay, social work expanded.

The 1905 Royal Commission

From the late 1880s, these two movements joined battle over the future of the Poor Law. This culminated in a Royal Commission in 1905 that was called to investigate the organization and operation of poor relief; it reported in 1909. In the ensuing controversy the Commission split between a majority (the COS) in favour of modifying the Poor Law, and a minority (the Fabians and their supporters) who favoured thorough reform (see Table 2.3). The Majority Report argued for a modification of the harsher aspects of the individualist approach to poverty, claiming that although self-caused poverty was a crime, deterring the poor was ethically and practically impossible. As Harris (1993, p. 240) remarks: 'Social policy towards public dependents should be "preventative, curative and restorative" rather than crudely deterrent.'

Table 2.3 COS and Fabian approaches to the poor

	COS view	*Fabian view*
Problem	Poor character	Inefficient organization of society
Organization	Modify Poor Law	Create new local authorities
Intervention	Selective/Individual	Universal/comprehensive

The Minority Report argued against the continuance of the role of philanthropy within the Poor Law. Far better to break up the system and require locally elected authorities to be responsible for the poor in education, childcare and health, leaving the unemployed to be dealt with nationally by central government. It proposed a degree of compulsion by suggesting that those not meeting the accepted standards of behaviour would be 'helped', whether they wished it or not. To police these new services, officials would be employed by the local authority to train and educate those falling from acceptable standards of behaviour. These developments had parallels with proposals sixty years later in the Seebohm Report (1968).

By the beginning of the twentieth century, social workers were attached to the many state institutions that had developed to deal with social problems such as poverty, sickness and old age. As Clarke (1993) argues, various voluntary organizations had workers linked to these institutions, thus providing a bridge between the inmates of such places and their immediate community. Lady almoners were employed to assess patients' ability to pay for treatment within the voluntary hospitals, and to provide assistance to the patient's family and relatives. Voluntary workers, known as court missionaries, attached themselves to the courts; they provided a service to those convicted and to the courts, by vouching for the character of the accused and offering supervision in the community as an alternative to prison. From these voluntary beginnings, state institutions then employed professionals to fulfil this role.

The findings of the Royal Commission in 1909 showed that the old Poor Law mentality had been dealt a severe but not a terminal blow. Across the political parties, including the Labour Party formed in 1906, there was a recognition that the state should take responsibility for certain aspects of an individual's welfare and progress social reform. Reform would not necessarily be informed by a developed social conscience; for example, the Conservative Party saw social reform as:

- a means to improve the efficiency and effectiveness of working people in the factory or at war
- a necessary evil to ward off social unrest and revolution.

Neither would there be unanimity between how much social reform should be pursued, but reform was none the less on the agenda. Thus a very basic old age pension and limited forms of health and unemployment insurance were put in place prior to the outbreak of the First World War. Where there was less progression was in how to treat those groups of people who were permanently removed from the labour market or who may experience longer spells of unemployment, i.e. those groups who would be reliant on the existing Poor Law. Although it was agreed by those social reformers involved in the Royal Commission that to revert to the overtly deterrent approach of the Poor Law was impracticable, the experience of those forced to rely upon it was different.

The inter-war years

Social work became detached from such wider questions of social reform by failing to develop its institutional base within the state. Between 1900 and the Second World War, although piecemeal improvements were made where the collectivist assumptions developed by the New Liberals and the Fabians gained ground, social work grew little in the state sector. The continuing expansion in the voluntary sector was directed towards families in poverty and was largely imbued with the philosophy of the COS. However, there were alternatives to the individualization of poverty; for example, George Lansbury and other members of the Labour Party in London worked particularly in Poplar to ameliorate the condition of the poor at a local level, by becoming elected on to the Board of Guardians to operate a more humane system of poor relief (Thane 1996). Conditions within the world economy were such that the late 1920s and the decade of the 1930s saw persistent and high rates of unemployment which meant that the inadequte systems of social insurance were unable to prevent large numbers of the unemployed from falling back upon means-tested social assistance. Throughout the 1930s unemployment remained consistently over 10 per cent of the total workforce peaking at 22 per cent of the insured workforce in 1933. For those forced to claim social assistance the future was bleak. Glyn and Oxborrow (1976) showed that an unemployed couple with three children would require £2.56 a week to meet their human needs, while unemployed assistance at that time was £2.10. The harshness of the Poor Law and the regime of public and unemployed assistance were to be powerful reminders for working-class people when it came for them to vote on a future government following the Second World War.

Although the hold of social work within the state was tenuous, its knowledge base grew and was influenced by the importation of psychoanalytical concepts from the USA. These ideas were used in the training of psychiatric social workers, and helped develop a specific area of expertise. The growth of expertise in the analysis and classification of personal problems was an important step in moving beyond the investigation and moral exhortation of the poor. The COS had already shown the importance it had placed on training in casework, and this was undoubtedly augmented by the developing science of psychology.

With this advance of knowledge came the recognition by government of its potential to control populations, especially those seen as troublesome to the social order (Foucault 1977). Social work took its place alongside medicine and psychiatry as an important source of strategic knowledge to control the conduct of persons. Social work knowledge referred to the nature of human beings and how they could be changed for the better, that is, for the improvement of wider society. Social work claimed an expertise that could analyse and predict human behaviour and, most importantly, rehabilitate persons back into 'normal' society. It was part of a 'normalizing process', in which the power of the state could be exercised through such techniques to control and modify the unacceptable traits of the destitute and the dangerous.

The post-war period

The impact of the Second World War

The Second World War and the subsequent election of a Labour government provided the social and political impetus to develop state welfare. The war highlighted many deficiencies within the localized system of welfare as it affected working-class people, particularly children, through the experience of evacuation. The employment of social workers gradually increased within the medical and children's services as the impact of war disrupted existing social relationships and community networks.

The public, remembering the high rates of unemployment of the 1930s, looked forward towards the end of the war and the creation of a better society. This was symbolized by the publication in 1942 of the Beveridge Report, which laid the foundations for the post-war Welfare State. This report proposed:

- a comprehensive and universal system of national insurance
- a national health service
- state responsibility for maintaining full employment
- a system of family allowances.

It was assumed that the state should take a leading role in providing for the welfare of all its citizens and not just for the poorest. As a consequence of the Report:

- a national insurance scheme was introduced in 1946, which provided for pensions, unemployment insurance and new family allowances
- a national health service was established in 1948, and a National Assistance Act was passed that required local authorities to provide a welfare service for older and disabled people.

This was an important moment for many who had so despised and campaigned against the old Poor Law. But although the Poor Law had been abolished in name, change was slow. The post-war Labour government put much effort into establishing a universal Welfare State, but did not include the PSS. It took a scandal, with echoes of current events, to compel the government to reappraise children's services and eventually reorganize them.

In 1945, Denis O'Neill, a child in care, was murdered by his foster-parent Richard Gough on a farm in Shropshire. Wartime evacuation had focused public attention on the problems of children living away from home. The Monckton Report that looked into the circumstances of the case found considerable neglect from the local authorities, which had supervised the child's placement. This criticism, coupled with the existing inquiry into children's services by the Curtis Committee, brought about the Children Act of 1948.

The two documents proposed that a personal and individualized service for children should replace the previous one, which had been characterized by bureaucratic indifference and administrative muddle. The Monckton Committee argued for recruiting more trained workers, who should be graduates with a social science training. The Curtis Committee agreed, proposing appropriate training to support the new children's service which it wanted set up. Curtis argued for courses for residential staff, and higher education training for the boarding out visitors who were to supervise the arrangements for placing children in foster care and adoption. Training should be monitored by a Central Training Council in Child Care. The Curtis Committee was open to the idea of making a complete break with the pre-war system, and called for a transformation in children's services. True to the post-war climate, Curtis called for change to be implemented by a state agency, 'which would energetically reform services for children, and infuse them with an entirely new spirit' (Jordan 1984, p. 74).

The ensuing Children Act 1948 laid down that:

- the Home Office should take policy responsibility for children's services
- the Children's Committees of local authorities were to be responsible for delivery of services

- children coming into the care of the local authority were to be assessed in residential centres to decide on appropriate action.

Personal social services followed this trend; local authority services were spread across a number of committees each with their own separate responsibilities. There were children's committees and health and welfare committees responsible for older people and people with disabilities. Not surprisingly, services became fragmented as each committee worked to their own organizational agendas. This made the co-ordination of services difficult. As Sullivan (1996) notes, the residue of the Poor Law remained in many of these services, as their low level of resourcing was reflected in the poor quality of buildings and inadequately trained staff.

The Children Act 1948 was a prime example. The assessment, in a reception centre, of children taken into care was intended to lead to placement in a family-type children's home, or with foster-parents; sadly this did not materialize. Instead, children were invariably housed in large residential establishments, where the promise of appropriate care in the community faltered. This was similar to the care made available by local authorities for older people in previous Poor Law facilities. Thomas Powell Roberts was born in 1915 and describes his experience of Ruthin workhouse's diet in 1940:

> For our dinner, we would have soup and rice pudding three times a week; two slices of bread, about one inch thick with a little scrape of margarine. We would have egg once a year at Easter. Meat occasionally – mainly fat with vegetables. No cakes and no sweets.
>
> (Roberts 1992, p. 16)

The period between 1948 and 1976 is often described as a golden age for the Welfare State, since spending on welfare services expanded at a considerable rate as the economy recovered. Social expenditure in the UK in 1960 was 12 per cent of gross domestic product; by 1976 this had increased to 19.6 per cent. The PSS missed out on this opportunity, and only in the 1960s did expenditure increase. The Conservative government, concerned with rising rates of juvenile delinquency and increased numbers of older and disabled people in institutional care, directed more resources to the PSS. Despite this, problems for the PSS continued with the fragmentation and poor co-ordination of services. Criticism from social workers and local government, coupled with the concern of a new government, provided an opportunity for review.

In 1965, the Labour government called the Seebohm Committee to review the PSS. The Seebohm Report argued that the PSS should be universalist in kind, not restricting itself to the most disadvantaged, but extending provision to the whole community. Seebohm talked about the need for universal services that would be community based, to explore the root cause of many of the problems experienced by the clients of social services. Since these problems were not necessarily individually caused, but were structural, society and its organization as much as individuals should be the target of intervention. Social workers would intervene within local services to ensure that their clients' entitlements were met. Any difficulties in the provision of and access to services would be dealt with, while the focus upon the individual's functioning in society would be maintained. The social worker was to initiate change within the social welfare organizations which were failing the clients of the PSS.

The Seebohm Report intended to make the PSS the fifth social service, a strong local authority-based department with resources and political power. It recommended the following:

- Each local authority would have its own unified social service department, to break down the fragmentation of service between the children's, health and welfare committees.
- Each local authority would have at its head a director of social services approved by central government. It was hoped that powerful new departments would become part of the local network of services alongside, for example, education and housing.
- Generic training should be developed for social workers, so that they could combine a variety of skills and experience within generic social work teams.

The expectation that reform would provide a unified and well-resourced service was to be unfulfilled almost as the new social work departments were instituted. As departments reorganized, large shortfalls in services were uncovered as previously excluded groups made their claims felt. These new demands arose at the beginning of a world economic crisis, which resulted in the government clawing back some of the resources earmarked for the new departments. Between 1970 and 1974 increased spending on the new personal social services averaged 12 per cent per year, but by 1975 the increase slowed to 3 per cent as the economic problems of the country were translated into reduced public spending.

Conservative policy

By 1979, a newly elected Conservative Party was promising further reductions in public expenditure and state responsibility for welfare. The arguments within the Conservative Party were enthusiastic in restoring the ideals of independence and individualism, echoing the Poor Law philosophy. A polemical book written at the beginning of the 1970s by one of the New Right's most vociferous supporters Rhodes Boyson (*Down with the Poor* (1971)) outlined this return.

> A state which does for its citizens what they can do for themselves is an evil state; and a state which removes all choice and responsibility from its people and makes them like broiler hens will create the irresponsible society.
>
> (from Clarke *et al.* 1987, p. 133)

In respect of the PSS the new administration called upon the Barclay Committee to review the roles and tasks of social work. The committee had no legislative brief but developed a number of recommendations that questioned the dominance of local authorities in delivering personal social services. The report called upon social work to be less ambitious and to prioritize the demands made upon it. This was in contrast to the hopeful recommendations of Seebohm only twelve years before. The main recommendations of Barclay were:

- closer involvement with the private and voluntary sectors;
- developing the role of social workers as enablers, working within community networks;

- development of community social work;
- closer links with the informal sector to reduce need for formal services.

Of more interest for social work and its future were the two dissenting minority reports that tried to pull Barclay in opposite directions, as shown below. Brown *et al.* called for a greater focus upon neighbourhood work, while Pinker was thoroughly sceptical about community social work.

The case for neighbourhood work

- Broad support for Barclay's community approach.
- Social work to relate to smaller units of the population.
- Focus on neighbourhood and 'patch working'.
- PSS to devolve its organization, greater decentralization.
- Mobilize community participation in PSS organization.
- Work more closely with informal networks.

(Based on Brown *et al.* in Barclay 1982)

The case against neighbourhood work

- Community social work based upon unproven assumptions.
- Community is a myth.
- Community social work will compromise the quality of social work.
- It will divert attention away from traditional casework, counselling.
- Traditional casework proven to work.

(Based on Pinker in Barclay 1982)

Barclay attempted a compromise between the burgeoning philosophy of the New Right and the old Seebohm vision of state-based social services. As such it both pleased and frustrated the Left and Right in equal measure. For the Right, the prospect of a reduced role for state services and the encouragement of the private and voluntary sectors was to be encouraged. For some on the Left, the idea of closer links with the community through devolved ways of working was attractive in developing greater community participation. As the economic problems of the British economy continued into the 1980s, the Barclay Report sank from view; the Conservatives had more pressing priorities to consider. The Conservative government was determined to withdraw state support for welfare through reductions in public expenditure. This was more apparent than real. Conservative rhetoric was indeed radical, but their actions were less so. The Conservatives introduced more radical legislation concerning the Welfare State, and in particular the PSS, in the late 1980s as their power base was secured in the House of Commons.

The Conservatives initially shied away from thorough, ongoing reform, yet some clues as to future policy were discernible. The White Paper, *Growing Older* (1981), outlined the future role for public authorities *vis-à-vis* the informal and voluntary sectors. They were to 'sustain and, where necessary develop – but never displace – such support and care' (DHSS 1981, p. 3).

The focus upon community responsibility was reinforced by Patrick Jenkin, Secretary of State for Social Services, who marked out the distance between the old Seebohm conception of the PSS and his own. The PSS should act as a safety net 'for people for whom there is no other, not a first port of call' (quoted in Sullivan 1996, p. 201). There followed in the early 1980s an overt encouragement of the voluntary and private sector, coupled with support for community-based social work initiatives, particularly in community care with adults. Grants to the voluntary sector were increased and the rules allowing the subsidy of private residential care through the social security system were relaxed. This resulted in spending by social security upon the private residential sector rising from a small base in 1979 of £10 million, to a formidable £459 million by 1986.

By the mid-1980s the Conservatives were beginning to flesh out their approach to the PSS; in a speech to the Joint Social Services Conference at Buxton in 1984 Norman Fowler outlined this vision.

- The PSS should have a strategic role and plan to take into account all the sources of care in the community.
- The direct provision of services is only part of the local pattern.

- The major role of the PSS should be in promoting and supporting other sources of care from the private and voluntary sector.

(Parton 1991, p. 211)

This view reinforced the notion that the PSS should be developing a mixed economy of care: the state was one of a number of providers of care in the community, together with the voluntary, private and informal sectors. Welfare Pluralism, as it became known, was an attractive option for the Conservatives. It could be used to erode state provision, while at the same time develop what they considered to be both morally and economically better alternatives. In moral terms it enabled family, friends and local neighbourhoods to care, increased independence and choice. It encouraged voluntary activity spontaneously, by removing the heavy hand of the state, so that people chose to help their family and friends because of their sense of responsibility to one another. This was far superior, it was argued, to the provision of impersonal state care and the removal of choice by the decisions of social workers.

In economic terms, the private sector was welcomed as superior because it used resources more efficiently than the PSS (see Chapter 6). This argument masked the increased burden that would be placed upon families, and particularly women within them, to care for their relatives. It also overlooked the fact that the lower operating costs of the private residential sector were achieved at the expense of employees, with wages and working conditions that were generally inferior to those offered by the local authority.

The Conservatives developed one conception of welfare pluralism, in which the PSS would be a residual service. It was to be a safety net, not for when the other arms of the Welfare State had failed, but for when family, community and the market failed. The Conservative Party wanted to develop the private provision of care and, so it was argued by their more radical ideologues, the private financing of welfare as well. By the late 1980s the Conservative government was ready to restructure the PSS; the changes envisaged were a reflection of their own ideological commitments and the increasing criticism by professional bodies and the public as to the inadequacy of community care services (see Chapter 5).

Conclusion

This chapter has charted the development of the PSS in relation to two influential ideologies, the New Right and Fabianism. Emphasizing the importance of the New Right in developing a tentative approach to social work in the early 1980s has set the scene for the more radical transformation of the PSS considered in later chapters. Significantly, the enthusiasm for a Fabian solution to the problems of the PSS as exemplified by the Seebohm Report was remarkably short-lived when faced with the profound economic and social problems of the 1970s.

Key points

- The study of ideology is essential in understanding the development of social work.
- Fabian and New Right ideologies have been key influences in the development of social work.
- Social work owed its beginning to the Poor Law 1834, and the COS in 1869, particularly in distinguishing the deserving from the undeserving poor.
- The PSS as the 'fifth social service' has remained a poor relation relative to other Welfare State services.
- From the early 1980s, social work moved towards developing a mixed economy of care.

Guide to further reading

Clarke, J., Cochrane, A. and Smart, C. (1987) *Ideologies of Welfare: From Dreams to Disillusion*, London: Hutchinson, is an excellent introduction that uses contemporary sources to describe the historical development and analysis of welfare ideologies. Sullivan, M. (1996) *The Development of the British Welfare State*, Hemel Hempstead: Prentice Hall/Harvester Wheatsheaf, provides a useful chapter on the PSS. George, V. and Wilding, P. (1994) *Welfare and Ideology*, Hemel Hempstead: Harvester Wheatsheaf, provides a thorough survey of the main ideologies informing the Welfare State.

Chapter 3

Anti-discriminatory practice and social exclusion

OUTLINE
This chapter will:

- outline the relationship between social exclusion and social work
- describe the links between anti-discriminatory practice, social work and equal opportunities
- discuss difference, diversity and social division as they influence social work
- describe the impact of social divisions in relation to social exclusion and social work.

Social work in a divided society

Britain is becoming an increasingly unequal society. Recent evidence shows that poor families are benefiting from rising standards in schools and falling unemployment but this has not altered corresponding inequalities in income or health. In respect to poverty defined as those living in households with less than half the average income, the proportion of children living in poverty, for example, has risen from 10 per cent in 1979 to 32.9 per cent in 1995–1996. These figures are exacerbated when we consider ethnicity, for example, 81.1 per cent of Bangladeshi children live in poverty. When family type and employment is taken into consideration 89.1 per cent of children living with a lone parent who is not working live in poverty (Adelman and Bradshaw 1999).

Over recent years, particularly since the mid-1990s, a new term has emerged to describe the process by which people become impoverished and socially marginalized, i.e. social exclusion. This concept was first adopted within the European Union and has become increasingly used in the UK. It is a useful term which involves an understanding of the social processes which lead to the marginalization of certain groups in society (Williams 1998). These social processes can be understood as:

● Relative in that they are concerned with how social relations create conditions of exclusion rather than individual circumstance.

● Involves action in which people are excluded by what others do to them.

● Movement over time in which social exclusion is dynamic, i.e. it may be transmitted from one generation to the next, or that persons may experience exclusion at particular times in their life cycle.

A recent study (Gordon *et al.* 2000) highlights this process in distinguishing four dimensions of exclusion. They are:

1 exclusion from adequate income or resources
2 labour market exclusion
3 service exclusion
4 exclusion from social relations.

These dimensions interact with one another, for example, labour market exclusion remains an important risk factor for both service exclusion and exclusion from social relations. For social workers, understanding the impact of social exclusion upon service users is central to anti-discriminatory practice (ADP). For example, exclusion from social relations, i.e. social isolation, is related to major caring responsibilities and to disability. Nearly 11 per cent of the population have very poor personal support available in times of need (Gordon *et al.* 2000). Thus certain excluded groups of people like carers or disabled people will rely more heavily upon social work and social care services for practical and social support when they need it. A focus upon social relations is important in that exclusion may be associated with poverty but is not necessarily the same. For example, the experience of gay men and women in rural areas led many to experience discrimination and isolation where the lack of social networks creates a heightened sense of their own exclusion. Similarly the isolation of people with mental health problems is reinforced by lack of adequate services and networks often coupled with outright hostility and lack of understanding (Pugh 2000).

Table 3.1 Indicators of social exclusion

Exclusion from adequate income or resources
- 60% of Pakistanis and Bangladeshis live in poverty and are more likely to live in a deprived area.
- Half of all disabled people have incomes below half the general population mean (usually taken as indicator of poverty).

Exclusion from labour market
- 2 million long-term workless households, number consistent since 1995.
- 50% lone parents without paid work.

Service exclusion
- Black Caribbean pupils are more than four times likely to be permanently excluded as white pupils.
- Over 40% of households without a care in rural areas say their public transport is bad compared with 12 per cent living in large towns.

Exclusion from social relations
- Women aged 60 or over are twice as likely to feel unsafe out at night than men.
- 300,000 pensioner households do not have a telephone.

Social exclusion is therefore a valuable concept to help social workers understand the processes by which service users require material and social support, yet there are a number of different understandings of social exclusion which need to be appreciated as they will influence policy responses to the excluded. Levitas (1998) identifies three such policy approaches in countering social exclusion:

- moral underclass
- social integrationist
- redistributionist.

Moral underclass

Emphasis is placed upon a permanently excluded residual population characterized by poor commitment to majority values of work and family; benefit dependent. Policy reduces incentives to stay on welfare benefits, and introduces penalties for anti-social behaviour.

Social integrationist

Argues that there are groups who have become temporarily excluded from opportunities in society, for example, those people made unemployed as industry restructures towards a service and technological industrial base. This perspective highlights the importance of work, training and education as the means to achieve social inclusion for those who have been unable to adapt to the demands of a global economic system. This view has been closely associated with New Labour (see Chapter 8). Thus the excluded must be socially integrated into society, where policy develops social opportunities for education and training to enable inclusion.

Redistributionist

Highlights the importance of reducing social exclusion by a radical redistribution of income and wealth to the poorest. Inequality which has increased over the past twenty-five years drives exclusion and must be a priority for policy.

The present government has set itself the target of reducing social exclusion and has set up its own unit (Social Exclusion Unit) to co-ordinate the government's approach. It seeks to mobilize all relevant government and local authority services to develop strategies which will focus upon particular groups who experience social exclusion; examples of groups who have already been targeted are rough sleepers and care leavers. For example, rough sleepers (Social Exclusion Unit 2000) are associated with misuse of drugs, mental illness, alcohol and poor or non-existent health care, leading to mortality rates twenty-five times the national average. Thus the government's strategy is to combine health, housing and training opportunities to remove people from the streets; social exclusion is multifaceted in that 'joined up problems require joined up solutions'. However, the government's approach has been subject to much criticism in that it targets specific 'problem' populations and then subjects them to an array of interventions in which the subjects of intervention have little or no control over what is done to them (Jordan and Jordan 2000). Levitas (1998) argues that New Labour's approach is heavily influenced by an integrationist approach which places too much emphasis upon work as a means to combat social exclusion when for many excluded groups it is the nature of the economic system (i.e. capitalism) which excludes them permanently whether in work or out of it. Social workers may also feel that this emphasis upon work also excludes many service users who are unable at this present time to achieve social inclusion through work and require immediate improvements in their current living conditions and capacities to enjoy a valued life.

Social exclusion as the product of increased inequality of income and wealth requires social workers to practise in a way that gives voice to the excluded by enabling an active citizenship. Social workers are in a unique position in that they work with the most disadvantaged and excluded people and can use their experience of working in partnership with individuals and their communities to have an effective input into influencing the agenda on social exclusion. This means that social workers engage with local community and self-help groups to enable both practical help and political engagement to counter processes of exclusion. This process implies that social workers will have to decide how they and their employing agencies can best use their limited resources to engage with and counter the reality of service users' exclusion (Lister 1998).

From radical social work to anti-discriminatory practice

By the 1990s, radical social work had been absorbed into the wider concept of anti-discriminatory practice (ADP). The idea of difference is crucial to this approach, which recognizes that reducing analysis to a single cause, such as class, can hide important areas of oppression. People are located differently in society as a result of race, age, disability, sexuality and gender. Older people (those over

65 years old), for example, make up 13 per cent of the total population of this country (Central Statistical Office 2000), yet wield little political power. Critics writing on ageism argue that older people are propelled into dependency, created by policies of retirement and inadequate pension provision. Older people are often seen as redundant and of little productive use for the economy once they have reached retirement age (Wilson 2000). Yet to explain the experiences of people from a single perspective, i.e. age, hides the diversity within that category. Acknowledging diversity as a concept permits a more sophisticated analysis, so that other social divisions, such as class, gender and race, will contribute to and influence the way that age is experienced and understood.

The diversity of people's backgrounds will have real consequences for their experience of the social work service they receive; issues such as gender and race influence the quality and quantity of service they are likely to receive. As Hughes and Mtezuka (1992, p. 222) remark, critical of the way some feminist writers have ignored age:

> Focus on these issues has not been balanced by an interest in older women themselves, either in terms of their experiences as recipients of care, or in relation to the strategies that older women adopt to meet the challenges of ageism and sexism.

The appreciation which social workers bring to difference and diversity influences their intervention with users. It can enable them to challenge the way the PSS reflect and reinforce social divisions in the delivery and organization of services.

The experience of marginalized groups in this respect may be described as 'dualism'; the case of black people in Britain is a useful example. Black people often experience insensitivity in the delivery of supportive services by the PSS yet are over-represented in intervention that involves the controlling aspects of social work. Chand (2000), reviewing research on child protection and black families, suggests black children are disproportionately represented at all levels of the childcare system. He outlines a number of critical factors, for example:

- poor interpreting services
- inadequate training of social workers
- misunderstanding cultural differences in child rearing.

Yet black families are more likely to experience unemployment, poor housing and minimal education than are white families and this requires preventive work by social workers. Despite the recent importance given to family support (Department of Health 1998) it remains that black children find themselves more likely to end up in care than their white counterparts. Preventive work requires social workers to build confidence and trust with black families but they are poorly prepared and supported to achieve this, as Chand suggests.

Social work and equal opportunities

The recognition that race and gender divisions pervade British society found its official expression in the development of social legislation in the 1960s and 1970s. The legislation concerning gender (the Sex Discrimination Act 1975 (SDA 1975)) and race (the Race Relations Act 1976 (RRA 1976)) reflected that formally, Britain ought to develop a society based on equality of opportunity. The individual and institutional barriers erected to deny women and black people access to employment and income was seen as denying the social right to participate as an equal member of British society. This was reflected in campaigns by women's groups, the trade unions and black groups to lobby for a legislative response. The advance of such social rights to fair employment practices and equal pay for equal work would, it was argued, counteract the discrimination met by many women and black people in the labour market. Two bodies were set up to monitor and address discrimination by sex and gender, the Council for Racial Equality (CRE) under the RRA 1976, and the Equal Opportunities Commission (EOC) under the SDA 1975.

The RRA 1976 made it illegal to discriminate directly in the areas of employment, housing, and in the provision of goods and services to the public. The CRE can take firms to industrial tribunal or court for cases of discrimination. For example, the Ford Motor Company's transport section was acted against in 1997. It recruited mostly from existing white employees, or the drivers' families and friends, so excluding applications from black and Asian workers in other sections of the Ford workforce.

The Equal Pay Act 1970 (EPA 1970) and the SDA 1975 brought in similar legislation for women. The EPA 1970 made it illegal to pay women less than men for doing the same work. The 1975 legislation made it illegal to treat a woman less favourably for employment purposes on grounds of gender. The EOC was set up to ensure that the law was enforced.

Both the CRE and the EOC have had some success, particularly in developing codes of practice to encourage best employment policy. They have been valuable in mobilizing opinion and acting as a focus for campaigning work in these areas. Unfortunately, both bodies have been limited by a lack of government funding and hostility from the courts in promoting the rights of groups over that of individuals. The Race Relations Amendment Act 2000 has made some important revisions to existing policy. This legislation owes its existence to the Macpherson Enquiry and the efforts of the campaign which investigated the murder of Stephen Lawrence by white youths. It extended the scope of the legislation to include the police, local authorities, the NHS and prisons, and now places the burden of proof of a fair racial policy on to the institutions which are charged with discrimination.

Recently there has been some extension of equal opportunities legislation towards disabled people and some extension of the rights of gays and lesbians in respect of the armed forces. However, a recent legislative development which may hold out opportunities for the future is the Human Rights Act (1998), for example, Article 14 appears to contain an absolute ban on discrimination, thus operating rationing procedures through arbitrary age criteria may well be open to challenge. Article 3 refers to inhuman or degrading treatment; therefore poor standards of care within children's homes or overtly punitive regimes of care again may be open to challenge. However, as Schwehr (2001) argues, the rights and freedoms contained in the legislation are not open-ended and require the courts to balance the interests of society against the interests of the complainant. Thus in regard to age restrictions for services a local authority may successfully argue that the additional costs of removing these restrictions may limit the extent of services for all older people.

Equal opportunities, social work and exclusion

Social work and social care services' response to exclusion is crucial in improving the lives of service users. This section outlines the different ways in which the social divisions of race, gender, age, disability, sexuality and class impact upon the lives of service users and reinforces their social exclusion. In focusing upon these divisions we are concentrating on single aspects of division, for example, gender refers to the social expectations about the behaviour of men and women. However, it is women who will experience greater exclusion and inequality from society than men. This relates to the different access to power and resources that men have over women, creating women as subordinate. These relationships of power and subordination have similar effects in relation to race and in other social divisions where relationships of superiority and subordination of one group over another are reinforced. This section focuses on those groups which experience social division as one of subordination. Crucial to redressing inequalities of power and resource in society are policies of equality of opportunity within social work and social care, and this has been translated into developing anti-discriminatory practice.

Race

Little work was done on the needs of ethnic minorities in the early years of the Seebohm reorganization; administrative concerns took precedence in attempting to make the new departments work for the population in general. However, the negative experience of many black people in the Welfare State was being voiced. Coard (1971) was highly critical of the education system, highlighting the over-representation of West Indian pupils in special units and special schools, and showed that this was a result of direct and indirect racism. Studies of racial discrimination in employment also demonstrated the deep-seated discriminatory practices of employers (Brown 1984). It was not until the late 1970s that social service departments recognized a problem in services for black people; a joint report by the Association of Directors of Social Services and the CRE (1980) listed:

- the low take-up of services
- the lack of employment opportunities in the PSS
- the focus upon general need overlooked particular needs of ethnic minorities
- the difficulty of developing appropriate services without extra funding.

The report argued that without extra resources to meet ethnic minority need, little could be done. In effect, the needs of these groups were considered as extra to mainstream service provision rather than being integral to them. The response of the PSS to demands for appropriate services may be characterized in three ways, as shown in Table 3.2.

Table 3.2 Types of PSS response to service demands

	Monoculturalism	Cultural pluralism	Direct racism
Treatment	sameness	cultural difference	cultural indifference
Service delivery	homogeneous	cultural adaptation	culturally insensitive
Service structure	white dominant	black marginalized	black excluded

Source: Adapted from Patel 1990; Rooney 1987

None of these responses deals with the expressed needs of the black community. Although a cultural pluralist approach, for example, recognizes cultural difference, it does not lead to the integrated delivery of service, but adapts existing service provision or adds on particular elements. This is done by offering a specialized service delivered by specialist workers (for example, a separate meals-on-wheels service serving halal prepared meals). This, in turn, leads to black services existing on the periphery of white-dominated service provision. Such marginalization has resulted in the black community developing voluntary responses to offset the shortfall in mainstream services; as Law (1996) argues, much of the work in defining need and making services more accessible has been done by black communities themselves. Recent developments in community care reflect the lack of urgency in developing policy in this area. The NHSCCA 1990 makes little mention of developing accessible services for black people. The proper recognition and assessment of the needs of black people are central to this process, as is encouragement to use appropriate services. Best Value under the Local Government Act 1999 has been used to at least require local authorities to recognize gender and race when assessing needs of service users. The evidence is not positive in regard to the recognition of ethnic minority need, since the Social Services Inspectorate/Audit Commission (1998) has shown that on average only around one-third of people who identified themselves as having such needs reported that they were taken into account in their assessment or in the services they received. These and similar findings led the Joint Review Team (2000, p. 34) to comment that:

> Generally, however, the picture is that black and minority ethnic service users lack the range of services appropriate to their religious and cultural needs and interpreting services are often inadequte for the needs of the community.

The black community remains sceptical as to the progress the PSS has made. This is well placed when, for example, a survey (of ninety-two PSS departments) showed that, while 90 per cent had an equal opportunities policy, including a statement on race discrimination, only 54 per cent had equal opportunities policies covering service delivery (Butt 1994).

Gender

Women form the majority of users and workers within the PSS. They make up 85 per cent of the total workforce, yet women are largely absent from managerial positions in the organization. At senior management level, assistant divisional director level and above, 18 per cent were women (Davis 1996). More men at basic social work grade are found within child protection, where career opportunities are greater, yet men are almost invisible within social care in the community. Women are better represented at managerial level in work with older people, but this carries less status.

Women carry out the bulk of the direct work with clients at all levels of the PSS. It is interesting to compare children's and adult residential care. The development of children's services after the Second World War attempted to provide smaller scale 'family type' accommodation. In these homes, staff were expected to model an ideal of family life, as reflected in the titles of staff as house-mothers and house-fathers. In the 1950s and 1960s pay was poor in residential care, and men were few. As pay and conditions improved in the 1970s, so men were attracted into the work. This was evident in the larger observation and assessment homes where the chances of career progression were greater.

By comparison, work with older people was the domain of women. Social work assessments of older people are biased towards practical caring issues, and work is short term, with little intervention designed to develop an older person's potential for change and personal growth. Work in the sector is seen as relatively low-skilled, and therefore the domain of women.

The kinds of services men receive compared to women is subject to gender discrimination. For example, men enter residential care at an earlier age and in better physical shape than women; when at home they tend to receive more domiciliary services than women (Hughes and Mtezuka 1992). These differences reflect the gendered assumptions regarding the respective abilities of men and women to care for themselves (see Chapter 6).

Disability

Many people with disabilities are prevented from exercising their basic autonomy. The freedom of movement to associate with others is denied through restrictive social environments. In the past, disabled people have effectively been shut away, either in large-scale institutions, or within their own or their families' homes and denied the opportunity to take their place in society. These barriers reinforce the assumption that people with disabilities are biologically and physiologically inferior to so-called able people.

Disabled people are described as being dependent, requiring them to be cared for; currently this is best achieved within the community. Morris (1993) argues that the provision of care implies the dependence of disabled people, who have to be cared for in the community, rather than enabling autonomy for an independent life. These assumptions assume a medical model of disability; disabled people are seen as cases to be treated, rather than as citizens with rights. Medical values have been central in developing the understanding of disability as loss or impairment. Disability, the argument runs, should be treated to restore damaged minds and bodies to as near 'normality' as possible. This assumption of 'normality' for the individual can manifest itself in direct medical intervention to fit a person into the 'normal' world, for example, fitting cochlea implants to develop hearing for children who have hearing disabilities. It can also manifest itself in exclusionary social attitudes, for example, to issues of sexuality. Disabled women often highlight this in relation to accepted stereotypes around women's sexual activity and attractiveness. Disabled women are seen as asexual, their attractiveness as impaired, and as having little concern in expressing their sexuality.

The medical model, by focusing upon the individual's impairment rather than the social environment, treats the disabled person as the problem. The critique of a society that creates barriers and disabling conditions for disabled people forms the basis for an alternative view. Writers from a disability perspective have turned the medical model on its head, arguing that it is the disabling social environment which needs to change, not the individual disabled person (Barnes *et al.* 1999). From this, a social analysis of disability has developed, emphasizing that disabled people can act for themselves in changing existing professional and societal definitions of disability.

In the area of employment, the current medical model gives grants to employers to adapt parts of their working environment for the specific needs of individual employees. In contrast, the social model argues for the general construction of a working environment open to all employees. Blakemore and Drake (1996, p. 156) argue as follows:

It entails the redesign, reframing, reconstruction and reconstitution of work through inclusionary policies, and work itself requires redefinition to encompass all people of all abilities.

Table 3.3 Models of service delivery and service disability

	Medical model	Social model
Service	Compensatory	Empowerment
Assessment	Assesses impairment	Assesses barriers to ordinary living
Examples		
Community care	Care-based	Independent living
Transport	Specialist/separate	Adapted into mainstream service
Employment	Individual grants to employers	General adaptation of working environment

The Disabled Persons Act 1986 was intended to improve the assessment, representation and consultation of people with disabilities, while charging local authorities with improving service co-ordination. However, the Act has not been fully implemented, and is silent on how it can be enforced if local authorities do not respond. This legislation, like others dealing with disabled people, is an example of government failure to give legislative power to deter non-compliance.

Discrimination in employment is a major issue for disabled people. The Disabled Persons (Employment) Act 1944 required all major employers (those employing twenty staff or more) to operate a quota system for people with disabilities. The quota was set at 3 per cent of the employer's workforce, yet 80 per cent of employers fail to meet this requirement. Even more striking is the fact that only ten prosecutions have ever been brought under this Act (Blakemore and Drake 1996). This has led the disability movement to call for more effective legislation, in what can only be considered as a matter of human rights. Calls for a Disability Commission with similar powers to that of the CRE and EOC have finally been met as part of The Disability (Discrimination) Act 1996 (DDA 1996). However, this legislation suffers in the most part from the same permissive approach to disabled persons' rights as has previous equal opportunities legislation. Disabled persons are given rights to access employment, and transport and other services, yet the responsibility for proving discrimination remains with the complainant and not with the organization complained against.

The DDA 1996 provides a limited advance for disabled people and will require social workers to use the provisions of the act to argue for inclusive services and opportunities for their service users. Much revolves around what are considered to be 'reasonable adjustments' that organizations have to meet in order to enable the needs of disabled people; thus social workers may be able to use their role as mediators and facilititators to argue that such steps are met without recourse to the law which is both costly and time consuming.

Age

This section will address the problems of age discrimination for older people rather than discrimination faced by younger people, which will be covered in Chapter 6. Although old age eventually affects almost everyone, little recognition has been given to addressing age discrimination. Employers regularly discriminate in favour of younger people in advertisements for work. More general changes in the labour market have encouraged older workers to apply for early retirement or to take redundancy packages offered by their employers. Current responses from governments and employers recognize the problem of ageism, particularly within employment, but little has been done.

Within the PSS a hierarchy of services places children as a priority over adults. Services for children have addressed not only the practical care of young people, but also their general developmental needs. Older people's needs, on the other hand, are generally seen as being physical in nature, with the assumption that inputs of service will need to increase with age. The implication is that older people will become a burden upon the resources of society as their numbers increase. Projections for the UK show that the percentage of those over age 65 was 15.8 per cent; by 2025 this is expected to rise to 19 per cent (Giarchi and Abbott 1997). Spending on older people is likely to rise, as increasing old age is associated with greater physical disability (particularly at age 75 plus). Yet as Wilson (2000) argues, this is not automatic as longer life will have a minimal impact, and most spending on health care is concentrated into the last two years of a person's life. Equally, many older people, rather than being dependent upon social services, are involved as care givers.

The problem of old age is therefore not necessarily one of age, but of the response of social policy towards older people. Pensioners comprise the biggest group: 41 per cent of those on means tested benefits in the UK (Howarth *et al.* 1999); the large numbers of older people living in poverty are testimony to the inadequacy of social security policies; older people in this country have below-average incomes compared to France, Germany, Belgium and the Netherlands (Phillipson 1998).

Policy towards older people has attempted to create financial security through developing full employment and social insurance. Thus the state provides a universal old age pension based upon social insurance, while encouraging workers to take out their own private pensions or employers to develop their own schemes to supplement state provision. Where this is not possible the Labour government has developed the idea of stakeholder pensions, which are designed to provide a top-up to the basic pension for those workers who are unable to fund their own scheme or who have no access to an employer's scheme. This scheme however will require a greater level of contributions for new entrants into the labour market than the previous SERPS scheme, and will be administered not by the state but by the insurance industry. Currently the state contributes 60 per cent of the total towards pensions and the individual 40 per cent; by 2025 the goal is that this will be reversed, placing a greater burden on the individual to fund their own pension.

The possibilities for older people have changed as better diet and living conditions shift current conceptions of old age. This can bring fresh opportunities for older people to break away from oppressive ideas of dependency, and for social work to respond in a positive way. Early retirement deals and relatively generous pension packages have increased the wealth and income, and therefore the spending power, of some groups of older people. These changes have led to lucrative business opportunities for firms within a niche market of affluent older people, the numbers of whom, however, are relatively small measured against the remainder, who continue to live in poverty. The economic value of older people, enhanced by these new consumption patterns, remains as long as they are relatively active, healthy and capable of spending their income. Conservative policy was successful for this affluent group, combining minimum state income with subsidies for private and occupational pensions to bolster incomes of relatively young, newly retired people. Social policy is more problematic for those groups with no access to private or employers' pensions, and to those older groups who need forms of care and support by others. For example, differences in what those at the top of the labour market can earn in retirement income is stark compared with those at the bottom. Lord Hollick (Director of United News and Media Group) can expect a pension of £9,200 per week compared to the current means-tested minimum income guarantee which the government requires a pensioner to claim of £91 per week (*Guardian*, 17 March 2001)

Community care policy is a useful example of the problems faced by older people. The dominance of local authority services has been steadily eroded by the development of voluntary and private alternatives. Although social workers as care managers control the service response to older people, there is less reliance upon residential options, and a greater emphasis upon keeping older people at home (see Chapter 6). This has some advantages for older people, since social workers, as the gatekeepers to the system, should prevent any arbitrary removal of those requiring financial assistance into residential care. However, the general development of community care may be no more welcome than the previous focus on residential care. The prioritizing of social work assessments means that older people will only receive an assessment, and consequently some services, if they have high support needs.

The General Household Survey (George 1996) found, for example, that there was a huge shortfall in practical help: some 33 per cent of people over the age of 65 required help in dealing with personal affairs, yet only 5 per cent were receiving any help. Social work with older people endeavours to maintain their presence in the community, yet this may not reduce the dependency experienced by older people. It is debatable whether an older person isolated in their own home with little social contact is any less dependent than a person in a residential home.

Sexuality

Sexuality as an area of study for social policy and social work is relatively new (Cosis-Brown 1998), yet its impact has been profound. Earlier social policies focused upon the perceived threats to society from certain marginalized groups if their sexuality and their potential to procreate were not controlled. People labelled as 'idiots', 'imbeciles' and 'moral defectives' (usually young women who had a child outside marriage) were confined to institutions as a result of the Mental Deficiency Act 1913. This Act attempted to segregate groups of people who were considered to have deficient intellectual and emotional capacity. This 'deficiency' was understood to be passed from one generation to the next; in order to reduce the possibility of the population to be 'infected', the ability of these 'defects' to have children should be curtailed. This eugenicist policy is echoed in recent cases in which some women with learning disabilities have been sterilized by medical interventions sanctioned through the courts.

The particular needs of gay and lesbian users have also been ignored, as has been evident in work with families. Their relationships are analysed as aberrations from a heterosexual norm. Gay and lesbian couples wishing to be parents are therefore a problem for the PSS that has often seen itself as a 'family service' (see Chapter 6). The 'ideal family' has invariably been interpreted as a mother and father having a conventional sexual relationship. The children of some lesbian mothers, for example, have been put into care; while older lesbians have been ignored when a partner dies, although appropriate social work support could have been provided (Cosis-Brown 1998).

These issues are also relevant to gay men and their wish to develop satisfying relationships with their partners, and to care for children. Gay men are often stereotyped; they are seen as sexual deviants who have a malevolent influence upon children and therefore may sexually abuse them. Evidence in relation to child abuse shows that it is heterosexual males who abuse young children, whether sexually or physically.

These concerns around gay and lesbian orientation have been felt in the policy over fostering and adoption; in 1997, Scottish fostering law made it impossible for gays and lesbians to foster children. In England and Wales, changes to adoption procedures in 1997 focused upon a 'common-sense' approach to adoption that would prevent social workers from making 'politically correct' decisions regarding the placement of children. This calls for more representation of parents with experience of adoption on adoption panels to decide on potential adoptive parents. The anxiety which restrictive policy promotes around adoption mitigates against a constructive and non-prejudicial assessment of the debate. Cosis-Brown (1998), summarizing research into parenting by gay and lesbians, 'shows no significant differences for children growing up in heterosexual or homosexual households in terms of risk or . . . social development' (p. 95). Of concern for gay and lesbian groups was the Conservative government's introduction of Section 28 of the Local Government Act 1988 which prevented local authorities from 'promoting' homosexuality. This has made it difficult to teach children in schools about the variety of sexual preferences in a balanced way, and has narrowed sex education to teaching about reproduction, marriage and heterosexuality.

If homosexuality is dealt with, it is often pathologized or seen as something from which young people should be protected. The present government, after making a pledge to remove this legislation, is now dragging its feet and it is unlikely that this will be repealed in the near future. Although Section 28 is practically dead through lack of legislative will it remains a powerful symbol of a homophobic society which seeks to suppress gay and lesbian lifestyles. This policy has been used to promote a particular view of the family and the appropriate behaviour that should take place within it. In making sense of these pressures, social workers are having to make informed decisions that should, in the case of adoption, for example, reflect a sober judgement about the capacities of adults to parent, and the appropriateness of particular families to look after the children placed with them. Consequently, prospective parents should, as Cosis-Brown (1998) argues, be subject to a thorough assessment as to their suitability. This means that accepting appropriate lesbian and gay carers may be as equally in the best interests of the child as refusing inappropriate heterosexual carers.

Class and 'underclass'

Anti-discriminatory practice, in engaging with the many dimensions of oppression, moved beyond radical social work's early privileging of class. In the debate on the complexity of social division, it can be forgotten that class remains a pervasive influence on the life chances of an individual. Class analysis has undergone a welcome renaissance in recent years particularly in relation to welfare policy (Lavalette and Mooney 2000) largely as a result of the persistence of class-based inequalities; for example, the Acheson Report (Acheson 1998) recorded continuing class-based disparities in mortality and for every major disease.

The term 'class' has many meanings, but will be used here to describe the structures of material inequality usually understood in terms of income and occupation. Income and occupation are appropriate indicators of class in mapping the 'material advantage and disadvantage in modern societies' (Crompton 1993, p. 10). In current capitalist societies, access to work and the income derived from it determines the quality of life for the majority. Social workers work with those in society who are largely denied this opportunity, or do so under conditions of increasing inferiority to those more advantaged in the labour market.

People on the edges of the labour market are likely to experience multiple disadvantages – unemployment, poor housing, ill health, disability and poverty. Social workers will tend to work with the poor in crumbling inner-city areas, or in the so-called 'sink estates' on the outskirts of the city or town. These areas are marked as qualitatively different urban spaces, characterized by rented accommodation, either from the local authority or increasingly from a local housing association, with a lack of local amenities, such as shops and adequate childcare facilities. In these communities, the schools will be low in the league tables of examination results, the students are likely to have low morale, and there will be high rates of absence and truancy. Here it will be impossible to get credit from official sources to help in buying essential consumer goods. These are places of social deprivation where the residents are in effect permanently excluded from the rest of society.

Some commentators claim that the bottom 30 per cent of persons by income are becoming permanently set adrift from the majority and are forming an 'underclass'. This group has been the target for recent social policy initiatives that have sought to force people back into the labour market. The New Deal, for example, targets groups which are said to form an underclass such as single mothers and the long-term unemployed and is increasingly requiring that claimants undertake education, training and work experience as a condition of their receiving jobseekers' allowance. Writers from the USA, such as Murray (1994), or the UK, such as Field (1989), have suggested that an 'underclass' has formed following the American experience. This group may be recognized by:

- rising illegitimate births
- a rise in violent crime
- permanent retreat from the labour market.

Murray's argument, though cavalier with the use of 'facts' (Morris 1994), is reminiscent of Victorian attitudes in which the underclass was seen as a physical and moral threat to society. Indeed, he characterizes the 'underclass' as a 'New Rabble' of single, morally corrupt individuals permanently adrift from a respectable middle class. This division, oriented around traditional notions of morality and the nuclear family, is increasingly adopted by the middle class, who are described as the 'New Victorians'. This view is supported by Dennis and Erdos (1992) and Dennis (1993), who argue that growing numbers of single mothers and absent fathers cause a variety of social problems within previously 'respectable' working class housing estates.

The validity of the underclass thesis may be questioned in respect of two key arguments:

 1 Arguments based upon different values
    A study of single mothers (Edwards and Duncan 1997) found
    that they held views which mirrored dominant views about
    appropriate forms of motherhood; a study of benefit claimants
    by Dean and Taylor-Gooby (1992) found little difference in atti-
    tudes to work, benefits and employment from the wider society.
    Thus the contention that there exists a group of people with dis-
    tinctly different values to the rest of the population is on shaky
    ground.
 2 Arguments based upon different behaviour
    Brown (1990), for example, argues against Murray's contention
    that an existing underclass is due in part to the increasing
    number of never-married mothers gathered in particular neigh-
    bourhoods dependent on state benefit. As Brown argues:

 • dependence upon state benefit is greater for divorced mothers than the never-married
 • the time never-married women remain so is limited as the
   majority eventually marry
 • the concentration of never-married in certain areas is a
   result of local authority housing policies allocating high-
   priority housing cases to the harder-to-let properties.

As noted above, the choices and behaviour of single mothers are
due to discriminatory housing policies and a lack of childcare facilities to facilitate paid work. Likewise single mothers choose in the
long run to remarry or live in long-term stable partnerships.

The debate regarding the underclass shows that there is a strong
constituency which prefers to blame the poor for their own condition rather than oppose the structural forces which result in
unemployment, poor housing and ill health. New Labour's
approach to social exclusion, dominated as it is by inclusion
through paid work has echoes of an individualist approach in
which it is the actions of the unemployed that are crucial to their
gaining employment rather than the operation of an unequal
labour market. Social work has always been involved with people
who are poor and socially excluded and who may not have access to
paid work; it remains for social workers to actively counter such
individualizing and discriminatory processes through their own

practice. Although resources to counteract poverty and exclusion are limited within the PSS social workers have an important role to play in counteracting social exclusion. Powell (2001) argues that social work agencies should be involved in 'poverty proofing' i.e. assessing the impact of its policies, procedures and practices to see how they may reduce poverty and social exclusion. On a practical level Dowling (1998) outlines the resources which social workers may utilize in offsetting disadvantage; for example, through the use of Section 17 money as part of the Children Act 1989 to provide support for 'children in need'. The idea that the PSS can offset all the emotional and material costs incurred by certain individuals living in a strongly competitive capitalist society has never been a possibility, yet social workers can still use their powers over resources and their skills as mediators and advocates to limit the impact on service users of living in such a society.

Conclusion

This chapter has shown the links between social work, social exclusion and ADP. It has argued for the importance of difference and diversity for an understanding of social exclusion. Some common themes have been noted in relation to difference and the social divisions studied. The different and diverse needs that are expressed by these groups are now the subject of a healthy debate as to the best way for the PSS to respond. It has shown the importance of recognizing the diversity of social need of different groups in society and how these needs have had difficulty in gaining recognition from the PSS. In acknowledging the importance of ADP for countering social exclusion, it has opened up a possibility for future development in recognizing that effective social change must engage with the needs of all excluded groups in society.

Key points

- The PSS must mobilize its resources to combat poverty and social exclusion.
- Difference and diversity are key concepts in understanding ADP.

- Difference and diversity combine in often contradictory and complex ways.
- No one attribute of difference (e.g. class, gender, etc.) is of sole importance in understanding the processes of social exclusion.
- Difference has not always been met sensitively by the PSS.

Guide to further reading

Blakemore, K. and Drake, R. (1996) *Understanding Equal Opportunity Policies*, Hemel Hempstead: Prentice Hall/Harvester Wheatsheaf provides a useful introduction to equal opportunity policies. For specific reading on particular groups see Law, I. (1996) *Racism, Ethnicity and Social Policy*, Hemel Hempstead: Prentice Hall/Harvester Wheatsheaf, Oliver, M. and Barnes, C. (1998) *Disabled People and Social Policy: From Exclusion to Inclusion*, London: Longman, Charles, N. (2000) *Feminism, The State and Social Policy*, London: Macmillan. For a book that explores the links between social work and social exclusion, Barry, M. and Hallett, C. (1998) *Social Exclusion and Social Work*, Dorset: Russell House is worth exploring. For readers interested in the rural context of exclusion and social work Pugh, R. (2000) *Rural Social Work*, Dorset: Russell House is an invaluable introduction.

Chapter 4

Residential care: the last resort?

OUTLINE
This chapter considers:

- the origins and purposes of residential care
- its use to control 'deviant' populations
- the development of social policy towards children and older people in institutions
- the current position of residential care as it applies to older people, children and young people.

What is residential care?

Residential care provides permanent or occasional periods of care for people who can no longer live, or have difficulty in living, in their own homes. Day care, in comparison, provides brief periods of care from which individuals return to their own home or residential establishment. This chapter focuses exclusively on residential care, as it is a unique and often contested resource that therefore merits particular attention.

Although residential care is part of a continuum of care, it is important to recognize that many physical and social barriers exist between residential establishments and the wider community; this is true for users and staff alike. Many of the controversies around residential care concern:

For users:

- loss of liberty
- social stigma
- loss of autonomy
- depersonalization
- low material standards.

For staff:

- low status compared to field social work
- lack of training opportunities
- poor pay and working conditions
- poor management
- low morale.

Social policy towards residential care has failed to engage with the issues above reinforcing the view that institutional care is the last resort (Jack 1998). The trend in the UK has been to move away from large, imposing and geographically isolated residential institutions, yet the effect of living even in small, seemingly well-connected community establishments is problematic. When a person is unable to leave, where they have no choice, where conditions have to be lived through and tolerated, institutionalization and social distance follow. Separation from the community is an important aspect of residential care provision, in which critics see a lack of visibility and, potentially, accountability that can lead to abuse. As the Waterhouse enquiry (Corby 2000) showed, even relatively well-regarded establishments by the PSS can operate abusive regimes, which are largely hidden from the community and the social services management systems.

Are these aspects of institutions inevitable, or can humane social policies be developed which treat people with dignity and respect? Supporters of independent and integrated living in the community would say that these aspects are inevitable. They have highlighted many of the adverse consequences of developing residential care that can become dangerously institutionalized. Writers from a disability perspective are very critical of the way institutional care created dependence of disabled people (Barnes *et al.* 1999). Recent evidence of care regimes within children's homes is mixed, showing a reduction of institutionalization from the 1980s (Berridge and Brodie 1998), while Sinclair and Gibbs (1998) found both liberal and restrictive regimes in the homes they studied.

The focus on keeping people in their own homes, and the move towards independent living for different user groups, has also led to the questioning of current policy on community care. Some groups of carers, in particular, argue that inadequate funding of community care services leaves extremely vulnerable people open to abuse or attack from the community. This has led to some carer groups to call for the rebuilding of residential facilities, which can care for those deemed vulnerable in the community.

As noted in Chapter 2, the adequacy of residential care has often been questioned. This has been reflected in the implementation within the PSS of policy which treats residential work as the least preferred option. Residential work has consistently suffered from limited opportunities for training and career progression; in much of Europe by comparison all residential staff are qualified following three-year courses (Lane 2000). Despite its lower status, expenditure on residential care remains high, accounting for a significant proportion of total expenditure; for example, in 1998/1999 residential care on older people accounted for £2,940 billion out of a total of £4,910 billion, for children the respective figures were £2,290 billion and £3,850 billion (Hill 2000). Residential care has received significant funding within the PSS, representing a formidable investment by the state which is now increasingly placed within the private sector.

The origins of residential care

Residential care has often been used by those in power as a form of warehousing to maintain populations no longer considered economically or socially useful to society. Thus the workhouses in the nineteenth century developed as places where the 'impotent' poor (e.g. the sick or infirm elderly) were kept (see Chapter 2). It has also been used to contain troublesome populations who may, it is argued, threaten the stability of society if they are allowed to live in the community. In the nineteenth century, those deemed as inappropriate for the workhouses were gradually removed to more specific institutions, such as asylums for those with mental illnesses.

Children were gradually removed from the workhouse by various means, including emigration to the colonies of Canada and Australia, fostering out, or being placed in specialist facilities such as industrial schools. The Children and Young Persons Act 1933 placed a duty on local authorities to board children out with foster families, and also to regulate the voluntary homes, where some children were also placed (Frost and Stein 1989). From housing an undifferentiated mass of the poor within the workhouse, the state began to classify persons according to specific characteristics or problems. Professional experts such as doctors, social workers and social investigators used their expertise to control and classify the poor. It was assumed that some individuals would be reformable through these techniques and would therefore be capable of returning to wider society.

This process of surveillance and treatment became a characteristic feature of both large-scale institutions, such as the asylums, and the workhouse (Foucault 1977). Residential care became part of the process through which the state attempted to control the conduct of individuals, by classifying them as particular social problems which could be managed by appropriate forms of intervention. The role of professional experts and the employees of the emerging welfare institutions was to turn inmates into 'normal citizens'. If the subjects were not open to, or were beyond 'normalization', then warehousing them away from society was the preferred alternative. Inmates were separated and classified into categories by age or condition to live out their lives in specialist institutions such as asylums. Separate provision was created to prevent moral contamination. The dangers of mixing the young with the old, or men with women, were obvious to the Victorian mentality, which saw the risk of depravity existing where the morally inferior were incarcerated together.

It was the development of the Welfare State following the Second World War that ended the reality, but not the spirit, of the Poor Law. Once responsibility for the unemployed was taken over by central government (as a response to the high levels of unemployment in the 1930s), so the Poor Law became the response to the problems of old age, disability and ill health. Although it was clear that the inmates of the Poor Law workhouses could no longer be classified as undeserving, eligibility for care was restricted lest those who could afford to fend for themselves took advantage of the workhouse system. An emphasis on individual and family responsibility continued in case residential care encouraged dependency among the poor.

By the end of the Second World War, the Poor Law ceased and the legal and administrative responsibility for statutory residential care passed to local authority departments. Their main responsibilities were in the provision of residential care for children and older people, under the Children Act 1948 and the National Assistance Act 1948. There were differences in approach to children and older people, marked by the concern that was shown about housing children in large-scale institutions. Thus the developmental need of children to live as far as possible in family-type residential care, or within substitute families, was seen as crucial. Another critical difference was in the involvement of the voluntary sector, which had been a major provider of residential care after the Second World War (when 40 per cent of children were looked after away from home) and reflected the interests of child-saving organizations such as Barnardo's. No such concern was voiced regarding older people, who were assumed to become increasingly dependent as they aged. For those in particular without adequate income they would be housed in large unsuitable institutions inherited from the Poor Law (Phillipson 1998).

Residential care and older people

In comparison with children, there was little attempt following the Second World War to develop alternatives to residential care for older people. Just as the service for children was meant to follow a family model, so the development of residential care for older people tried to formulate a service approach to care. This model, taken from the private sector, was meant to show that residential services for older people would break with the Poor Law mentality by emphasizing the care and protection of older dependent people. Care centred on practical and health aspects, reflecting dominant medical assumptions that old age was a time of physical infirmity. Most employees were women, and their training, if they received any, was minimal, this state of affairs continues to the present day (Wilson 2000).

Until the 1960s, local authorities were slow to develop residential care for older people; much long-term care continued in former workhouse dormitories or former Poor Law hospitals in the health service. The influence of private care was minimal upon the state sector, although its service ethos was influential in the ideology of residential care at this time. The ideal was for the state to try and emulate what were considered to be the higher standards of care in the better private homes, which were seen to operate more as genteel hotels. The typical resident, if there was to be one, would require supervision and care, rather than have any particular chronic health need. Those with long-term health needs would be cared for in long-stay geriatric wards as the responsibility of the health service. However, boundary disputes between the PSS and the NHS were not uncommon over where responsibility lay for those older people who had less clearly defined health or social needs.

By the late 1960s, residential services for older people had fallen into disrepute. A number of highly critical studies showed the lack of respect and dignity afforded older people by health and social care staff; this was compounded by the lack of resources and the residue Poor Law mentality (Townsend 1964; Meacher 1972). Townsend's descriptions of the large wards and dormitories, where older people were confined with little stimulation or appropriate care, were damning. He argued that little had changed for older people since the end of the Poor Law. Meacher's book described how the needs and preferences of older people were in many cases ignored by their social workers and their families. The older person was literally taken for a ride and placed in permanent care with no prior knowledge or consultation. It was therefore not surprising that this evidence had a significant impact in fostering a negative view of the future possibilities of residential care for older people (Peace *et al.* 1997).

> People live communally, with a minimum of privacy, yet their relationships with each other are slender. Many subsist in a kind of defensive shell of isolation. . . . They are subtly oriented towards a system in which they submit to orderly routine, lack creative occupation. . . . The result for the individual seems fairly often to be a gradual process of depersonalisation.
>
> (Townsend 1964)

Criticism of residential care across all user groups stimulated much debate about the adequacy of training for residential services staff. This led to a general review of training, the Williams Report 1967, which was unique in that it considered training for all residential workers for the first time. It reported that the numbers of trained staff employed in the residential care of older people were minimal, and none were trained in social work. Nursing qualifications predominated within the state, voluntary and private sectors, but no full-time staff held recognized social work qualifications (Williams Report 1967).

Throughout this period, large variations in service could be observed with different local authorities providing significantly different levels of service. Whether an older person came into care often depended more on the lack of supportive services in the community than on any informed assessment of their needs. While research such as Townsend's encouraged debate, it had little impact at policy level due to local authorities' fear that older people would become a financial drain on the local community (see Chapter 3). This was reflected in the way older people were assessed. Assessments were often carried out by unqualified welfare assistants, whose main aim was to assess the older person's financial resources. Those entering care were means tested and their resources taken to make some contribution to the local authority. This is similar to the current assessment of older people under the National Health Service and Community Care Act 1990 (NHSCCA 1990) and which has led to much current debate (see Chapter 5).

By the 1980s, the problem of the increasing number of older people was placed centre stage, provoking the Conservative government's response *Growing Older* (1981). The debate focused upon cost. The state could not, it was argued, be involved in the expansion of residential care to meet the expected demand placed upon residential services by huge numbers of older people. By 1982, the state provision of residential care had reached its limit as resources were cut. English and Welsh authorities provided 42,900 residential places for older people in 1952, and by 1986 they reached their maximum in providing 124,300 places (Sinclair 1988). From this time, local authority care declined, as the Conservatives encouraged the private sector. This was rarely contested by the PSS or the NHS;

both were provided with a significant subsidy via the social security budget.

- The PSS could reduce its expenditure on residential provision and allow the private sector to grow.
- The NHS could gradually withdraw from its responsibility to provide continuing care, and transfer this to the PSS.

This resulted in a retreat from the NHS principle of free health care. Patients transferred into the community were subject to a means test for nursing and residential care. The NHS had been able to shift its responsibility so that continuing care was virtually a PSS responsibility; chronic (long-term) care was increasingly social care, while the NHS focused on acute (short-term) treatment. Despite the NHSCCA 1990 encouraging collaboration between the NHS and the PSS, conflict over the needs of patients – as to whether they needed health or social care – continued. Current arrangements under the Health and Social Care Act 2001 are proposing to integrate health and personal social services by pooling budgets and creating joint management systems around social care, and a new category of intermediate care will provide help for people immediately following or through a period of acute illness. These plans will give a greater role for the NHS in the provision of social care. These new arrangements may prevent the PSS and NHS from protecting their budgets by defining need in terms of the other's service – resulting in the so-called 'boundary wars'.

Although no general policy statement about older people and residential care emerged in the early 1980s, a policy was nonetheless being pursued. The Conservative government allowed older people to claim their fees for private residential care from social security (subject to a means test) if that care was deemed essential. Thus the private sector was allowed to expand through the public subsidy of social security payments (see Table 4.1).

The Conservative government attempted to manage this process by:

- putting a ceiling on the amount that the state would pay through social security
- regulating the quality of private provision through the Registered Homes Act 1984.

Table 4.1 Residential home care places (elderly, chronically ill
and disabled people) as a proportion of total places (%)

	Local authority	Independent sector
1970	63	37
1990	39	61
1998	22	78

However, these provisions neither contained costs in the private
sector nor did they lead to any significant increases in the quality of
the care provided. As Sinclair (1988, p. 277) pointed out: 'These
measures face the difficulty of simultaneously containing public
expenditure and ensuring high quality care.'

Paradoxically, the most important impact on residential services
for older people came from the developments that led to the
NHSCCA 1990. These changes, as is shown in Chapter 5, were to
put local authorities in charge of all assessments into residential
care that required state support. This put the budget formerly under
the control of social security into the hands of the PSS and,
although on the surface generous, many local authorities questioned its adequacy against a backdrop of tighter budgets from
central government.

The NHSCCA 1990 provided the impetus to restructure residential care for older people. Previous policy had implicitly
favoured the expansion of private residential care; the requirement
placed upon local authorities to spend 85 per cent of their new
funding in the private and voluntary sector made an explicit statement that the provision of local authority residential care was to be
a thing of the past. Since the early 1990s, there has been a rapid
decline in local authority residential care with an expansion of the
independent sector (voluntary and private).

The increasing provision of private care has also been met with a
corresponding response to push the cost of such future care on to
individuals rather than the state. Proposals by the previous
Conservative government to further privatize pensions and to
encourage pensioners to take out their own care insurance, through

a partnership plan with the government, would have increased the financial burden on older people. The Labour government instituted a Royal Commission on Long Term Care 1999 whose report did not meet with unanimous approval from the government. The key issue was the Commission's majority report recommendation that personal care and nursing care should be free of charge following a needs assessment but that housing and living costs should be paid for, while a minority report favoured maintaining means testing for residential care. The government favours the minority option in this case and has decided to keep a large element of means testing in the funding of long-term care, although it has accepted the argument for free NHS nursing care. The Labour government does not propose to alter the balance of provision delivered through the independent sector but prefers tighter regulation of the sector. The Care Standards Act 2000 creates an inspectorate replacing the PSS responsibility in this field with eight regional commissions for care standards who will monitor all care homes including local authorities for the first time, taking over regulatory responsibility from local authorities. A key feature will be the setting of national standards which will, it is argued, enforce minimum levels of provision that can be measured against agreed standards. This will be policed and enforced by the inspectorate.

In respect of the staffing of residential care there are a number of factors which may improve conditions. First, the setting up of a Care Council will require all care staff wherever they work to be appropriately trained and qualified. The introduction of the national minimum wage is also of importance here as at least staff pay will be tied to a statutory minimum level, although this is not generous. However, despite these improvements in general the current position on staff recruitment is not favourable. In the residential sector problems include:

- an ageing workforce – projected retirement higher than replacement rate
- 70 per cent of residential homes report recruitment problems
- decline in registration and awards for National Vocational Qualifications.

(SSI/Audit Commission 2000)

The private residential sector is now under pressure to provide more care with less funding. Local authorities argue that they cannot increase money for residential care as other demands for community care and children's services compete for resources; in addition, money from central government does not cover the full cost of meeting need in the residential care sector, leaving local authorities to meet the difference. This shortfall also impacts upon prospective residents who find that they or their families having to make up the shortfall in funding to stay in a home of their choice. The government's preferred option for older people is to provide more intensive support at home which requires greater additional costs than if older people went into the residential sector. This funding problem has led to the closure of private residential and nursing homes leading to a net loss of 9,700 places last year (Wheal 2001). The impact of the Care Standards Act 2000 is also significant as both local authority and independent homes will have to meet new standards of care which will push up costs again for this sector. The combined pressure of costs and raising standards of care is likely to lead to a greater rationalization of residential care leading to smaller economically inefficient providers, leaving the industry and the larger national and multinational companies to move into the sector (Player and Pollock 2001). This trend has been noted by Knapp *et al.* (2001) who show that as of January 2000 just eighteen large (mainly quoted) companies together operated 1,360 homes, approximately 22 per cent of all private sector UK provision. These corporate providers operate significantly larger sized homes averaging out at fifty-four beds per home compared to thirty-five in the local authority sector. These are worrying figures given the strong association of larger home size with poorer standards of care.

The future for residential care is likely to remain with the private and voluntary sectors, whatever political party is in power. The trend within the UK mirrors similar developments in Europe. In those countries where the state had previously taken responsibility for this provision, there is clear evidence that the provision of residential care is moving towards the private and voluntary sectors. For those countries which have previously emphasized the role of the independent sector, such as Germany, this trend is intensifying.

In the financing of such services the trend is towards self provisioning, i.e. individuals paying for their own services either directly through private insurance or through a mix of private insurance and public subsidy.

Residential care for children and young people

Residential care for young people has declined significantly in the UK since the 1970s, from 45,000 in 1975 to some 5,000 (Department of Health 1999b). It has been highly controversial, with enquiries and scandals highlighting the inappropriate and harmful 'care' provided in some residential establishments. Utting (1997) argues that the decline must be halted so that the children's home sector can provide real choices for children and young people in care. This view is challenged by those who argue that residential care is a costly and inappropriate option when improved foster care would be far more appropriate (Berridge 1997).

Table 4.2 Children looked after by placement (March 2000)

Fostered by relatives and foster parents	38,000
Children in local authority homes	5,000
Children living with parents	6,500
Children adopted	3,100
Children living independently	1,200
Other accommodation	4,200
Total	58,000

Source: Department of Health Local Authority Statistics 2000

The shift towards the community has its roots in the reforms of childcare services following the 1960s. Parker (1995) outlines these changes:

- the decline in funding voluntary sector provision and the transfer of resources into children's departments
- the move by the voluntary sector into prevention rather than residential services

- local authorities taking over responsibility for those children in approved schools (previously with the Home Office) through the 1969 Children and Young Persons Act
- removing distinctions between children in need of protection and young offenders to develop a preventive family service
- the reorganization of the PSS following the Seebohm Report into a unified and integrated service.

By the early 1970s, the numbers of children coming into care was falling. The overall number staying in care, however, was rising, as children stayed in care longer. Concern from the permanency movement suggested that little work was being done to prevent children from coming into care. To avert future problems, it was suggested that children needed to have a stable, permanent set of relationships upon which they could count, and that care should not result in children being moved from one placement to another. This was not translated into keeping children in their own homes; rather it meant that once the decision had been made to place a child in care, the child should be speedily placed into a situation of permanence. This often meant the swift removal of the child and finding a permanent adoptive home. This process was facilitated by the Children Act 1975, which gave local authorities the power to place children for adoption quicker than before. This was not met with universal support; arguments against the idea of permanence came from:

- the black community, who argued that permanence was inappropriate; the invariable placement of black and mixed-race children with white families denied these children's sense of racial identity
- those who viewed the approach as too punitive and condemnatory of working-class/ethnic minority parents, from whose children a disproportionate number were taken into care.

It was felt that permanence was an inappropriate response when more effective support could maintain children in their own homes (Parker 1995).

The increase in the number of children in care that followed the 1975 Act was politically unacceptable at a time when resources were cut back within the PSS. This gathered momentum with the 1979 Conservative government's determination to cut back on state expenditure and enforce greater reliance on individual and family responsibility. The numbers of children in care began to fall, and children's homes were sold off and closed; fostering and other community alternatives, such as community family centres, were promoted. As community alternatives were seen as the preferred option, the steady fall in the numbers of children in care in the 1980s paralleled the rise in the numbers of children on at-risk registers (see Chapter 6). Pressure to overhaul childcare practice intensified as a result of:

- disquiet at the rising numbers of children on at-risk registers
- a succession of critical child abuse enquiries
- research showing that the assessment and placement of children in care was the least preferred option.

The Department of Health (1991) confirmed this disquiet in its retrospective review of research:

> The well-being of children being cared for by social agencies is enhanced if they maintain links with parents and children. Unfortunately other research showed that all too often links were not maintained.
>
> (From Bilson and Barker 1995, p. 368)

The subsequent Children Act 1989 included a number of important changes for residential childcare stressing the importance of family ties in determining any prospective action regarding the placement of children. The main points were:

- It required local authorities to review existing childcare policy and re-examine their priorities in the light of the legislation.
- Section 34 of the Act introduced the idea of partnership between the local authority and parents to ensure reasonable contact.
- It introduced the idea of accommodation; children whose parents are temporarily unable to care for them would in the main be accommodated, leaving the parent(s) fully responsible for them.

(Bilson and Barker 1995, p. 368)

The reality of 'partnership' is not straightforward. It is important that contact with parents is maintained (as will be discussed below), but the same difficulties remain as to when to continue contact with parents and when to deny it. The best interests of the child may require prevention of contact with parents. The experience of partnership at the investigation stage has found that this process, as expected, is highly contested (Corby and Millar 1997). Parents have not, in general, agreed with social workers' decisions, and the statutory requirement to investigate and assess their families has produced confusion and disappointment.

Following the election of the Labour government, two important documents, *Quality Protects* (1998) and *Modernising Social Services* White Paper (1999a) have both emphasized the duty of local authorities as having a corporate responsibility for the welfare of children. This means every department of the local authority and not just the PSS. As a result local authorities have a number of objectives to meet which they must fulfil in planning children's services and are subject to penalties if they fail to deliver.

The impact of residential care upon children

In the early 1990s, a succession of reports (Kahan 1994) demonstrated a 'powerful consensus' in calling for:

- the end of the idea that residential care was 'second best'
- residential care as part of a planned and coherent framework of all children's services
- the need for proper management, inspection and monitoring of children's homes
- the need to value and train residential care staff.

These criticisms of the residential sector rather gloomily describe the low morale among staff and residents, and the feeling that residential care was set adrift from other areas of social service delivery and management. The subsequent reports of residential scandals did much to confirm the drift that had taken place in the management of residential care (Corby 2000). The reality for children is that many admissions into care are unplanned emergency responses to breakdowns either within their families or in other areas of the care system such as fostering.

Although figures are hard to collect, Simm (1995), who was a member of the residential care taskforce set up by the government to advise local authorities on residential care services, suggests that emergency admissions made up between 70 and 80 per cent of most receptions into care, and any figure under 50 per cent was rare.

The backgrounds of the children coming into care also play a part, as the vast majority are from homes characterized by poverty, often lacking the resources to alleviate potential crises. As Bebbington and Miles (1989) showed, of 2,500 children coming into care:

- three-quarters were living with a single parent
- almost three-quarters of their families received income support
- only one in five lived in owner-occupied housing
- over half were living in 'poor' neighbourhoods.

Bilson and Barker (1995) conducted research on the amount of contact children had with their parents and their social workers. Their research showed that the longer children stayed in care, the more likely they were to experience isolation, instability and poor parental contact. Bilson and Barker compared foster care with residential care and found there were significant differences in the children's experiences. They concluded that:

> Long periods of placement in foster care were associated with less parental contact whilst in residential care longer stays were, if anything, associated with higher proportions having parental contact.
>
> (Bilson and Barker 1995, p. 378)

This research confirmed previous findings (Stein and Carey 1986) that many children in care or accommodation could not expect stability of placement; as children grew older in the care system they were likely to experience greater instability.

The longer children stay in care, the less contact there is between social workers and parents. The possibility of partnership, unless addressed early on, is therefore likely to fade. The impact of isolation on children therefore further devalues residential care. This is compounded when increasing numbers of older children form the residential population, leaving this sector as the safety net for those who have been through community options such as foster care. These problems are often presented as evidence of failure, yet for some children there is no foreseeable alternative, as all other options in the community have been exhausted.

The present government's White Paper *Modernising Social Services* (1999a) is unequivocal in its condemnation of the care system which it says has abused and neglected children, but there is much to do. Not only are residential institutions already socially isolated from parents and social workers, but management of some homes has failed to address this problem. Jordan (1997), commenting on the many scandals around residential care in the early 1990s, shows how some of the problems share common themes:

- lack of external managerial control
- failure to implement new working practices, particularly in the light of the Children Act 1989
- senior management (often male) exercised authoritarian control, care staff (often female) felt intimidated and powerless to act
- no encouragement for training or development.

Social policies towards residential care have promoted it as a place of last resort, housing those young people with major social problems. Children come into care who have committed serious criminal offences or who have been victims of serious criminal offences. Estimates reported from residential staff suggest they believe that up to one-third of children have been sexually abused (Kahan 1994). Given the level of training and support residential workers receive, it is unlikely that they will find this manageable.

Some local authorities, such as Warwickshire and Lewisham, have responded to these dilemmas by closing down their children's homes. However, there is a price to be paid for such a move. In Warwickshire, an evaluation by the National Children's Bureau showed that the children experienced even greater instability as they were moved between foster carers who were unable to cope, or they ended up in residential care anyway, yet at a distance from their local community. As Simm (1995) argues, this policy was based on the assumption that there was a pool of foster carers waiting to care for children – but this was not the case: 'Many authorities saw their remaining provision operating almost in a state of siege, where whichever homes had vacancies had to take all comers' (Simm 1995, p. 17).

Despite the many problems faced by residential care, evidently some consumers of this service have benefited from it, and they have consistently argued for its retention. The National Association of Young People in Care (NAYPIC), for example, suggests that for some children it is the most preferred and beneficial option, stating this view in a variety of government enquiries into residential care for children. The immediate issue is the appropriate resourcing and support of such a service. A consultative document issued by the Department of Health (1999c) found, for example, that the proportion of young people leaving care at age 16 had increased from 33 per cent in 1993 to 46 per cent in 1998. They suggest that costs are a major factor in local authorities pushing children into the community but also suggest that children themselves are voting with their feet. If there continues to be a significant number of children requiring residential care then policy has to become more positive in valuing the sector as an essential resource for children. Jack (1998) reviews the ideological antipathy towards residential care as being one of the major barriers to the development of policy. Parker (1988) argues that it is not possible or desirable to close children's homes as each year his estimate is that some 3,000 places will be required largely because the foster care system requires an outlet for children who would require breaks from this provision or leave altogether.

Given the increase in child poverty (children are disproportionately represented in low income households: Howarth *et al.* 1999) and its strong association with residential care, children will continue to require safe residential provision. The failure to date of residential care is not something innate to residential homes but more to do with the management systems in place to ensure quality in care and adequate resourcing of homes. For example, the Waterhouse Enquiry mainly refers to the experience of large children's homes (sixty-plus residents) that were in place in the 1970s in North Wales when much of the abuse took place. Children's homes in the main are now much smaller, with residents typically in single figures (Corby 2000). Social policies that prescribe an enthusiastic adoption of community alternatives only for children in care per se run the risk of providing inappropriate forms of care for children and young people who would prefer more communal forms of care.

Leaving care

For young people, leaving care is a major life transition, yet the level of support they receive is not encouraging. Stein and Carey (1986) showed that children coming out of care are more likely to be unemployed, change accommodation frequently, and lack the necessary educational qualifications to prepare them for the outside world. Recent studies confirm this evidence. The Social Services Inspectorate (SSI 1997) acknowledged:

- three in four care leavers have no academic qualifications
- more than half become unemployed immediately.

The SSI also commented on the poor quality of services provided for care leavers and the variability of standards across the UK. Many care leavers are left largely on their own to cope with a major transition in their lives. To improve the situation, an integrated set of social policies that can plan, prepare and ultimately resource children's transition from care into the community is required. The government's Social Exclusion Unit has targeted children's transition from care as one of its priorities and has begun to take an integrated approach to the many problems experienced by such children. As a response to these initiatives the Children Leaving Care Act 2001 will supply ring-fenced funding to local authorities to provide better support for children coming up to and leaving care. This will mean that every 16-year-old in care will have a young person's adviser, there will be a personal pathway plan developed which should outline a strategy to plan for the young person leaving care and local authorities will be required to maintain contact with children for the immediate future once they have left care. It is an attempt to create a national strategy for transition. This is an important development which should provide improved support for care leavers and hopefully cut down on the number of children leaving care unsupported, or running away from care, given that between a quarter and one-third of rough sleepers have been in care at one time or another (Social Exclusion Unit 2000).

Conclusion

In this chapter we have discussed the development of residential care, emphasizing its roots in the Poor Law and the subsequent housing of troubled and troublesome populations in specific institutional settings. The provision of residential care for older people and for children and young people has been investigated and the differences in approach between the two noted. Residential care is often seen as highly damaging for younger people, while for older people it is often seen as an almost inevitable outcome of being old. Neither proposition can be said to be valid, considering the relative benefits that some children derive from residential care and the relative disadvantages that some older people continue to experience.

Key points

- Residential care is seen as a place of last resort.
- Social policy towards older people in residential care is influenced by considerations of economy.
- State residential care is likely to continue but be limited to those with higher support needs.
- Residential care for children and young people is an essential resource within the childcare system.
- Social policy towards child residential care must develop more positive responses which value this resource.

Guide to further reading

Despite its importance, there are few current books on the social policy of residential care for children or older people. Barbara Kahan's (1994) *Growing up in Groups*, London: NISW is a most comprehensive summary of residential care for children, which includes some social policy context and summaries of recent enquiries into residential care scandals. For a positive analysis of children's residential care, Crimmens, D. and Pitts, J. (2000) *Positive Residential Practice: Learning the Lessons of the 1990s*, Lyme Regis: Russell House, is a useful exploration of childcare in a residential context. For residential care in relation to older people, Peace, S., Kellaher, L. and Willcocks, D. (1997) *Re-evaluating Residential Care*, Buckingham: Open University Press, is a comprehensive account.

Chapter 5

Community care

OUTLINE
This chapter will:

- describe the development and concept of community care
- chart the decline in institutional care in the 1960s and 1970s
- describe the development of current community care legislation
- analyse the mixed economy of care
- describe the developing forms of managerial regulation.

What is community?

The concept of community has achieved new significance as a means to value social solidarity within a world which it is argued is increasingly fragmenting into individualism (Bell 1993). All the main political parties emphasize both the duty governments have to support communities, and the responsibilities citizens have to maintain them. These ideas have crystallized around the ideology of communitarianism (Etzioni 1993) which has generated a lively debate about its appropriateness for social policy. Communities, it is argued, should encourage positive behaviour by their members such as the development of trust and mutual support. These solidaristic behaviours, it is argued, form the basis of our interactions in families and local neighbourhoods, encouraging communities to support the unfortunate and condemn those seen as transgressing accepted standards of behaviour. Communitarian philosophy is particularly insistent upon the benefits of informal social control that communities can bring, yet this has its problems. The insistence on a moral solution to such problems as crime or social neglect clearly overlooks the importance of material constraints individuals and communities face which cannot be easily solved by moral exhortation (Hughes and Mooney 1998). New Labour has been influenced by communitarian principles and is particularly concerned in promoting its benefits in relation to the care of people within their own communities and to issues of crime (Johnson 1999).

Community therefore has great moral and practical significance pointing to the way we ought to relate to one another but also becoming the focus around which the PSS delivers services. Different definitions of 'community' have different implications for the organization and delivery of the PSS.

- *Community as a geographical concept denoting an area or neighbourhood*
  For example, the Barclay Report (1982) promoted the idea of 'patch working' with a team of social workers engaging within a locality, encouraging local care networks to develop a patchwork of local services.
- *Community of common interest/shared culture*
  This can cover a geographical area, for example, a religious community such as Muslims from Bangladesh who settled in large numbers within the London Borough of Tower Hamlets. However, common interests may not be located geographically, for example, gay communities may be geographically spread throughout a city or large area. The organization of supportive services may therefore have to take into account the geographical spread and the discrimination and stigma faced by such groups.
- *Community as shared networks of relationships*
  These may be over wider areas than geographical locality, implying that community is relational as well as geographical. The Griffiths Report (1988) assumed that families can provide readily available informal care, yet merely the distances which family members now live from one another can hinder this.

Although community is often thought of as invariably positive, it is not always so. Communities which define themselves in distinction to others create negative consequences for those which do not fit their definitions of normality. The assumptions underlying community care, for example, that people previously confined to institutions will be welcomed back into the community, are often belied by hostility from neighbours fearful of their property values if such groups settle near them. Similarly, newly arrived immigrants and asylum seekers, second and third generation black citizens continue to experience racism at the hands of some members of the white community. Communities can be hostile places for those seen as different, who may not fit narrow habitual expectations.

Communities are also divided along class lines; different communities may be exclusively divided through class, i.e. working and middle class, forging relationships within them in quite different ways. Thus working-class communities are often trapped in spaces over which they have little control. They may well develop supportive relationships within them; but they continually have to fight for resources to provide a social infrastructure of support. The middle classes experience community differently, as characterized by an advantageous spread of public and private amenities and services. Middle-class communities use their power to maintain privilege and distance from those seen as a threat to property values or labelled as undesirable in some way (Hughes and Mooney 1998). This results in reinforcing advantage for the middle class and requiring working-class communities to struggle for decent social environments.

History of community care

The observation that communities have always cared for their members on an informal basis has been used to argue that current community care policy is a natural development of the past. A critical examination of history questions this view. From before the Industrial Revolution until the early 1960s, people labelled as severely mentally or physically disabled were understood to be better cared for in long-stay institutions. The 1959 Mental Health Act began the drive to develop community care by:

- reducing the legal constraints on keeping individuals in psychiatric hospitals
- suggesting a major reduction in hospital beds for people with mental health and learning disabilities
- recommending an expansion in supportive community facilities.

This policy was unsuccessful; admission rates to large hospitals rose, while people moving into the community found that community care services were largely non-existent. In spite of the inadequacy of community services, by the mid-1960s a significant body of opinion was arguing against keeping large numbers of people in long-stay hospitals (Jack 1998). The record of long-stay hospitals had become tarnished by a series of scandals concerning vulnerable people kept in appaling conditions, such as in Ely Hospital in 1969. Although community support was in its infancy, there was great enthusiasm to rehabilitate people from these damaging environments. It was assumed, particularly by the social work profession, that resources saved from closing long-stay hospitals would be transferred to local authority community services.

The importance in developing community support, for example, around domiciliary care, assumed that the state should support the informal sector. Without the intervention of the state, families would be unable to bear the responsibilities of looking after their kin. Thus, to make community care successful, the state's role as a provider of services was crucial in reinforcing familial responsibility (Means and Smith 1998). By the late 1960s the government was taking a greater interest, particularly for people with mental health and learning disabilities; two White Papers (Department of Health and Social Security 1975a and b) proposed that local authorities would have the main responsibility for care and treatment. Sadly, enthusiasm for community care was hampered by a lack of strategic thinking. For example, the hospital service, which had the most resources, felt it could best develop community alternatives. The difficulties were in:

- developing clear lines of responsibility
- freeing resources locked into residential care in the NHS and the PSS
- determining where health care finished and social care began.

Both the NHS and the PSS had claims to make over the future allocation of community care resources, yet as Walker (1989, p. 207) comments, there was a 'lack of political determination to translate even the most minimalist policy into common practice'.

As a result, the supply of local supportive services continued to lag behind demand.

By the mid-1980s, Labour and Conservative governments had tried to unlock some of the resources stuck within health and PSS. The 1977 Joint Finance Initiative:

- made money available from health to fund community care initiatives
- speeded up the running down of hospitals
- diverted people in the community from entering hospital.

This was followed by the Community and Joint Finance Initiative 1983, which provided some £15 million to look at innovative ways of moving people from institutions into the community. Both initiatives explored imaginative ways of managing individuals' care within the community, and gave social workers flexibility in organizing packages of care by involving the informal and voluntary sectors. This reflected a shift in the conceptualization of community care: from care in the community to care by the community (see Table 5.1).

Table 5.1 From care *in* the community to care *by* the community

Care in the community	
Primary role	Provision by community health and personal social services
Secondary role	Supplementary neighbours, friends and family
Care by the community	
Primary role	Family, voluntary agencies and the private sector
Secondary role	Enabling by health and social services overseeing plurality of care provision

Although the Conservative government was firmly in favour of care by the community, its lack of a clear strategy to achieve this aim led to much criticism. The House of Commons Select Committee on the Social Services (HMSO 1985), for example, pointed out:

- the bias in some communities towards moving people out of hospitals
- the lack of recognition of the existing contribution of carers
- the lack of community support for carers
- the lack of what constituted 'good' community care
- the exhaustion of joint finance arrangements
- the lack of clear joint working arrangements between health and social services
- the small weight consumers' views had in the delivery of community care.

The Audit Commission (1986), which was the government's own investigative body, delivered its own critical analysis, observing that:

- Progress was slow in moving people from long-stay hospitals into the community.
- Resources did not follow former patients moved into the community.
- Perverse incentives (subsidy from social security payments) encouraged older people into residential care.
- Services were fragmented with inadequate staffing levels in community.

The government responded by asking the managing director of Sainsburys, Peter Griffiths, to look into the way public funds were used to support community care.

Community care and the Griffiths Report

By recommending changes in the organization of community care services, the Griffiths Report reinforced the intention of the Conservative government to change the role of the PSS. As Barnes (1997) argues, Griffiths placed the role of informal care centre stage alongside the development of the private sector. This strategy was, in effect, a process of dual privatization. Services were contracted out to the private and voluntary sectors, while the family was expected to make a greater contribution to care.

Griffiths' brief was to work within existing resource levels to comply with state expenditure targets. He makes this clear: 'To talk of policy in matters of care except in the context of available resources and timescales for action owes more to theology than to the purposeful delivery of a caring service' (Griffiths 1988, p. iv).

His recommendations, that the PSS and not the NHS has responsibility for community care, surprised the government. It was anathema to an administration that had a strong ideological resistance to local government, particularly Labour-controlled local government, and had done much to diminish its power. The proposals, however, implied a significant reduction of local authority provision of community care. Griffiths' key proposals were that local authorities should be 'enablers', organizing and directing community care. The private and voluntary sector should provide most care, which would be purchased by local authorities which would control community care funds transferred from social security and the NHS.

These recommendations signalled changes in financing and delivering community care services by local authorities. The core of Griffiths' proposals were adopted, but those which implied a greater role for the state and local authorities were dropped; for example, the proposal for a Minister for Community Care was also shelved. The government finally published its response in the White Paper *Caring for People* (DoH 1989), outlining six key objectives:

1 to enable people to stay at home where possible, by targeting domiciliary, day and respite services to those in greatest need
2 to give priority to the needs of carers; in assessing care needs, carer's family should be included
3 to tailor packages of care to individuals by giving priority to needs
4 to encourage maximum use of private and voluntary sectors in the provision of services
5 to make agencies accountable for their performance by clarifying and publishing their responsibilities
6 to secure value for money for the taxpayer by introducing new funding arrangements for social care.

The development of quasi-markets that would enable the inde-pendent sector to provide community care was central to the government's proposals.

Commentary

In theory, a quasi-market mimics an ordinary market in which buyers and sellers exchange goods. In a quasi-market there is a monopoly purchaser (the local authority) which buys community care from a number of providers (the sellers are the independent sector, or the local authorities in-house services). It is argued that this develops cost-efficient community care, of a standard acceptable to the local authority, by promoting competition between providers.

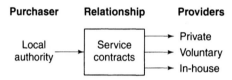

Figure 5.1   An example of a quasi-market

The subsequent NHSCCA 1990 required local authorities to spend 85 per cent of their community care funds in the independent sector. Local authorities would negotiate contracts with them for the provision of community care services. They would ensure that the standards for quality of services and care were met, through monitoring by their own inspection unit. It was planned that over time, local authorities would slowly withdraw from most provision of community care services. Many local authorities were enthusi-asts for the new arrangements; they argued that their role would be maintained through the development of quasi-markets. Central to this process was the role of local authorities as assessors of need who were required:

● to produce an annual community care plan setting out guide-lines and future objectives in partnership with health and other relevant community interests

- to ensure appropriate individual assessment of need, including
  the ability to pay for services, and to organize packages of care
  based on these individual assessments
- to develop care management to oversee the delivery of services.

The mixed economy and its consequences

The mixed economy of care is now well entrenched within the
PSS. Since the NHSCCA 1990 became fully operational in 1993
local authorities have continued to develop their relationships
with the independent sector. The imperative of value for money
remains foremost in planning and delivering services, and this has
been encouraged by New Labour which expects local authorities
to make year-on-year savings of some 3 per cent of their total
budget for the PSS. For the previous Conservative government
ideally the quasi-market in care was to be the generator of an
increasingly privatized service, for New Labour retaining contractual relationships between purchasers and providers is
necessary but not sufficient. Developing a strong regulatory
framework is crucial to limit the fragmentation and inequity
between local authorities that quasi-markets are prone to (DoH
1999a). At the core of this process is Best Value which sets key
performance criteria for the PSS to meet and from which year-on-
year improvement is expected. Local authorities can be disciplined
and face the threat of having the management of their services
taken over by outside bodies brought in by the government. As
part of this process a wider framework for measuring performance
has been introduced (DoH 1999b) which includes fifty performance indicators that can be used to compare local authorities'
performance across the range of PSS activity. The current government therefore retains quasi-markets but seeks to use them to
generate efficient services rather than develop particular forms of
independent provision as the Conservatives wished. Thus New
Labour is ambivalent about the form of community care
(public/private) but wishes to control what is being delivered,
focusing upon a regulatory framework to attempt effectiveness,
equity, efficiency, quality services and user empowerment
(Johnson 1999).

Table 5.2 Community care policy

Moving from	Moving towards
● Service-led assessment	● Needs-led assessment
● Public provision	● Mixed economy of provision
● Institutional care	● Home-based care
● Health provision	● Community provision

Modernization and community care

In analysing the proliferation of White Papers, guidelines and current legislation that concerns local government and the PSS, the key aspect of reform is one of 'modernization'. Fairclough (2000), writing on the language of New Labour, suggests that modernization is used almost exclusively in relation to welfare reform, while in relation to the PSS the connotation is unambiguous in suggesting that the PSS requires thoroughgoing transformation. *Modernising Social Services* (DoH 1999a) is explicit in its enthusiasm for modernization which it argues will deal with the failures of the past. These are:

Failure to protect

Vulnerable adults have been unprotected in the community leading to breakdowns in care and abuse.

Lack of co-ordination

In community care the NHS and the PSS have often been involved in arguing over whose responsibility a particular service user's problem is rather than addressing the issue itself.

Inflexibility

Service users' needs are often fitted into existing service provision rather than addressing what suits the service user.

Poor understanding of role

Service users, social workers, the public and social service managers often do not know which services should or can be provided and what standards of service should be expected.

Lack of consistency

There are large variations between different local authorities in relation to assessments of community care.

Inefficiency

Many local authorities can get better value for money for the services they provide; for example, in relation to charging for services.

These failures are not new and have been identified at the beginning of the chapter as endemic to the social and political context of community care (e.g. Audit Commission 1986). As Langan (2000) argues, this cataloguing of failure assumes that responsibility remains only with the PSS, while many of the problems identified above were beyond the control of the PSS; for example, government subsidies which saw the uncoordinated expansion of private residential care, or the hospital closure programme by the NHS in moving ex-patients into the community. The modernization process therefore builds upon the provisions of the NHSCCA 1990 and in particular confirms that this is a problem of management and seeks to refine this process. In the following section community care policy will be evaluated, particularly in the period up to the election of a Labour government, and its implications assessed for current policy. Following this an analysis of specific issues in relation to current managerial developments will be made to show how New Labour seeks to develop the process of managerial control and accountability further.

Evaluating community care policy

The aims of community care policy in the 1990s are summarized in Table 5.2 (p. 95).

Needs led

Local authorities are required to produce annual community care plans outlining their assessment of need in the community and their strategies to meet it. Care management was introduced to assess users' individual needs and develop packages of individual care. Many social work managers embraced these opportunities enthusiastically, arguing that innovative provision could be developed to break away from existing methods of delivering social services. Progress has been uneven. A number of user groups have tested local authorities' resolve to provide appropriate needs assessments and have shown that resources remain a fundamental problem. In March 1997, Age Concern lost an appeal (under the Chronically Sick and Disabled Persons Act 1970) in the House of Lords in which it argued that Gloucestershire County Council should not withdraw community care services on resource grounds only. The assessment of need has been compromised by the pressure to work within existing resource levels, leaving those with significant community care needs short of appropriate services.

This is not new – but inadequate resources diminish the concept of needs assessment. As Hirst (1997a, p. 10) has pointed out, across user groups in '70 per cent of metropolitan areas, over a quarter of those assessed end up with nothing at all'. These figures may be repeated for learning disabilities; for example, a study for Scope (Lamb and Layzell 1995) found that 87 per cent of those studied had not received a needs assessment. For those who had received an assessment the majority felt that their needs were inappropriately shoehorned into existing services. The variability of initial assessment has also been commented on by the Joint Review Team (2000) who have identified significant variations between local authorities who offer an assessment to virtually all service users referred to them and those who offer assessments to barely one-third referred to them.

In order to meet the shortfall between demand and supply for community care, local authorities have increasingly turned to charging for services. Government assessment of local authority needs through the Standard Spending Assessment already assumes that charges represent 9 per cent of their income. Thus in areas with overall levels of poverty, authorities which collect less than 9 per cent will experience an effective cut in their income from central government.

Charging has become increasingly important for local authorities, as a recent report by the Audit Commission (2000) in relation to home care outlines:

- ninety-four per cent of authorities now charge for home care compared with 72 per cent in 1992/93
- charges in one-third of councils can leave users with less to live on than the income support appropriate to their age
- users in similar circumstances but different areas face charges that vary from nothing to over £100 per week.

Thus the current government is concerned to create national frameworks which it is hoped will reduce unacceptable variations in charging. Charging is therefore now well entrenched within the PSS and the government seeks not to reduce the levels of charging for services but rather to manage them more effectively. As the Audit Commission (2000) makes clear, charges are an integral part of enabling councils to use them to extend access and improve services. This is worrying for those who would like to see charges limited in the PSS, as the assumption appears to be that better access and improvements in services can only be developed by indirect payment by the most vulnerable for the limited service they already receive. It is also problematic, as much research into charging shows that it denies access to services for the poorest clients, since they fear incurring the extra costs of services charged to them. Alcock and Pearson (1999) have also shown that those people who have to pay charges as their income is above the income support level (which most local authorities use as the cut-off point for charges) find that some service users' income then actually falls below the income support level. The above findings can be further developed; for example, disabled service users with a wider range of needs have found that the costs of paying for care take greater proportions of their income; this has increased anxiety, stress and the further risk of poverty (Chetwynd *et al.* 1996). Baldwin and Lunt (1996) in their review of charges found that local authorities were concerned that charging:

- reduced use of services
- increased financial hardship
- gave poorer quality of life for service users
- eroded relationships between service users and professionals.

Lymberry (1998) has concurred with the above findings and argues that the impact of the NHSCCA 1990 has been to create less flexible services with a greater focus upon procedural and managerial requirements of budgetary control. Ellis *et al.* (1999) concur with these findings in their research of assessment practices within community care social work teams, finding that those teams with the highest rates of referral were the least flexible, resorting to criteria-driven assessments reinforced by the use of new technology to manage their workloads. This has occurred at the expense of social workers' professional relationship with service users and has narrowed the ability of social workers to respond to the social needs of service users. This difficulty in responding to need by social workers has led to increasing frustration about the nature of care management which maximizes bureaucratic-driven tasks at the expense of social workers' skills (Postle 2000).

The mixed economy

The mixed economy if it is to operate at its optimum should:

- encourage communities to participate through informal care
- give choice to users of services
- encourage efficiency, effectiveness and economy of provision.

Informal care

Feminist writers on community care argue that the assumption of a fairly stable and available pool of informal carers is problematic and requires unmasking. Women are increasingly unavailable to provide care at home, as they expect to take their place in the public sphere of work; the participation of women in the workforce is steadily rising as men's is declining. Women working full time increased by one-fifth between 1984 and 1997; overall the number of available carers also decreased from 6.8 million in 1990 to 5.7

million in 1995, and some two-thirds of women are carers (Fawcett 2000). Issues of class, race and sexuality reinforce the diversity of experiences that women have of community care (see Chapter 3).

- Carers in lower social classes are more likely to experience ill health and disability and have fewer resources to access formal care.
- Working-class women carers under age 45 are more likely to provide co-resident care.
- Black women not only provide care at home but are forced into low-paid caring jobs, often in community care and health. In effect, black women become doubly exploited by the state through their formal (low pay) and informal (no pay) caring tasks.
- Gay and lesbian carers do not fit easily into the familial ideology behind caring; their relationships are often seen as illegitimate and lacking the 'permanency' of heterosexual couples. Their relationships are often characterized as 'pretend'.
- Gay or lesbian partners' status as next of kin remains unclear; for example, they will have difficulty in handling their partners' financial affairs or in signing consent for medical treatment.

(Cosis-Brown 1998)

The dominant assumption behind the mobilization of carers in the community is that carers are drawn from stereotypical families with little variation of relationships within them.

Choice for users

Choice for users depends upon a variety of flexible and responsive services which in a quasi-market compete for the patronage of the user. As noted above, with the increasing use of charging for services, choice has often been assumed to flow from the purchasing power of the service user as a consumer. For users to become consumers, they need to be able to choose the community care services they want. Thus users make choices by exiting one service they consider inappropriate and buying into an alternative. Service users can also act as citizens in demanding a voice in the development of services so that choice is exercised through a political decision-making process involving service users. New Labour has sought to encourage local authorities to consult in this way (see Chapter 7). Evidence suggests that users have little say in planning community care services, with great variations between local authorities. Wistow *et al.* (1996) found that only a minority of local authorities involved users in the planning and purchasing of services. Where consultation and participation has occurred, users and carers have largely felt positively that their views have been taken into account and acted upon (Barnes 1997).

Quasi-markets do not empower users as consumers; it is the care manager who takes on the role of consumer and decides upon the appropriate package of service, and controls the budget. The idea that users can be the direct consumers of services is illusory unless they have the financial means, but even here, problems remain. There are human and social limitations to choice. For example, consumer choice requires that a person makes judgements based upon their ability to act and choose rationally between alternatives. Yet for many service users they may be in a situation of crisis where their rationality may be compromised by ill health, stress and mental incapacity which creates significant barriers to rational choice.

A consumer model assumes that users themselves have control, for example, over their own spending on care; this is clearly available to a limited number of wealthy service users, but it is only with the Direct Payments Act 1996 that some element of user control of budgets has been introduced (see Chapter 7). Control over budgets is important, but involvement in the commissioning of contracts within the mixed economy can also increase choice of providers. However, direct local authority intervention in the market (to ensure that contracts are placed with those providers who will offer a service to meet their requirements) offsets this. As Henwood *et al.* (1996) observe, in order to ensure the quality and cost of care, local authorities may prefer block contracts, which will limit the number of competing providers and reduce choice. This effect has been evidenced by Andrews and Phillips (2000) who have shown the negative effect that this process of control has had on small residential homes, so limiting the scope of competition.

Although there has been much competition in the residential sector, the provision of independent domiciliary services has only recently grown to offer potential choice to users. As priority is given to those users with a wider range of needs, others lose out. Users who are considered to have minimum requirements are required to pay for their own care in the private sector, rather than choose between the local authority and an alternative.

Efficiency, effectiveness and economy

Developing the mixed economy of care and quasi-markets incurs additional monitoring and administration costs for local authorities. Increasing the numbers of managers and administrators is usually done at the expense of fewer staff delivering the front-line service. As services are more fragmented, management systems and bureaucracy increase to monitor the process, leading to delay, complexity and therefore costs; for example, £600 million for inspecting local authority services in 2001. Henwood *et al.* (1996, p.17) suggest similar problems in their study of five inner London boroughs: 'The price . . . has been shown to be a vast increase in bureaucracy as more forms feed burgeoning information and information technology systems.'

Means and Langan (1996) have also noted an increase in bureaucracy in relation to assessments and charging policies towards older people with dementia. They found that older people with a high level of need were caught up in complex bureaucratic procedures that hindered prompt and equitable treatment.

Home-based care

The experience of home-based care varies across society, according to class, gender, disability or cultural background. Morris' (1991) work on the needs of disabled women shows differences in what the community and the home mean for different women. She points out that some feminist literature sees developing community care as a product of an ideology that reinforces women's dependence (Dalley 1997). Many disabled women, whose independence is denied by institutional forms of care, view moves towards the community more positively if it leads to more control over their own lives.

In considering community care, preparation is required to make this transition successful, requiring co-ordination of different agencies to supply appropriate services. Progress has been slow in co-ordinating and developing a choice of living options, particularly for those seeking greater independence. The differences in perspective between some feminist writers and disabled women reflect the lack of flexible alternatives within community care. Feminists have always argued against community care because of its repressive consequences for women as carers. More flexible approaches to community care, based upon independent living principles, would free women both as carers and users from their forced dependency upon one another.

In prioritizing community care, financial considerations influence the assessment of home-based care. Local authorities will attempt to contain the costs of keeping a person at home by suggesting residential care when maintaining them in the community becomes more expensive. Local social service departments increasingly rely upon the local housing authority to provide suitable accommodation. Successful provision of home-based care depends upon the availability of appropriate and affordable housing; this invariably means rented housing. The Conservative government's encouragement of home ownership for council tenants depleted the existing stock of affordable rented property in the council sector. This means that although the proportion of 'special needs' housing in the public sector has risen, the overall level has not (Sapey 1995). In response to these problems the current government has attempted to provide more flexible ways of encouraging people to stay in their homes; for example, their proposal to allow a person entering residential care to avoid a financial assessment on their home for the first three months of residential care may allow a person to move back into the community and their own home if their situation improves.

Despite the fact that the NHSCCA 1990 recognized the need for local authorities to plan housing for people requiring community care, the majority of local authorities have done little to assess the housing need of disabled people. In organizing housing, local authorities now deal with a fragmented mixed economy of welfare, making more use of the private sector and housing associations. As a result planning and co-ordinating community care becomes more complex. Studies of housing need show that some local authorities make provision and develop innovatory projects, while the majority remain locked in responding to current need, rather than planning for the future (Watson and Harker 1993). To this end recent developments have attempted to co-ordinate the role of the PSS and housing organizations to enable the PSS to provide greater support through transferring money for special needs housing to the PSS. Likewise the new arrangements for intermediate care under the Health Act 2000 will provide free care for those people who may at present be too ill to return home but who in the longer term may be able to return once they are fitter.

Community provision

In moving services from hospitals, community planning arrangements are required to transfer resources and provide appropriate health and social care; the NHSCCA 1990 required health and social services to plan together. To be successful, community care requires collaboration between health and social services, which is difficult given the atmosphere of conflict and mistrust developed in the past. Community care legislation intended to provide a seamless service between health and the PSS, but this is yet to be achieved. Table 5.3 shows some of the key points of conflict.

Table 5.3 Areas of conflict between health services and personal social services

● Who is responsible?	● Discharge of people into the community
● Definition of needs	● Health or social care
● Conflict over priorities	● Low priority groups – substance abusers, people with disabilities?

Who is responsible?

These tensions have been recognized by New Labour which is attempting to overcome the boundary problems between health and the PSS; for example, the Health Act 2000 allows local health and social care bodies to find ways of integrating services. Recently the Health and Social Care Bill 2001 (going through Parliament as I write) gives government new powers to require local authorities and health bodies to pool their budgets where services are failing. Care Trusts will be created which would provide all the health and social care to a specified population. Wistow *et al.* (1996) suggested that some health and social services have made improvements in collaboration and joint commissioning. They cited the growing evidence of joint community care plans published and the development of working agreements between health and social service staff. Real success will be measured by how far social services and health share their resources through joint commissioning. This will be difficult, as both parties will have to commit resources towards joint projects, which in turn means losing control over some aspects of their respective services. It appears that the current government has therefore decided to force the pace on this issue and create a body under the auspices of the NHS. Many local authorities feel uncomfortable with this, seeing in the proposals the takeover of social care by the health service. The problem is that a service concerned with issues of ill health and treatment may not be best placed to deal with social care; this is one of the reasons why the previous government kept social care under the control of local government. In addition, a care trust does not have the same accountability to service users as local government through the democratic process of local elections, which may reduce its responsiveness to service users.

Definition of needs

Different organizational and professional approaches in the community before the NHSCCA 1990 gave rise to conflict over the definition of need. Users requiring a basic service were often fought over; for example, arbitrary distinctions were made between district nursing services and home care. This could reach ludicrous proportions: for example, whether a person was given a bath on medical or social grounds. Similarly, a social care worker may remind a person to take a particular prescribed medicine but may not administer it – a medical health worker has to do that. The development of working agreements defining who is involved in health and social care has been one of the advantages of the recent legislation. However, as resources become tighter these disputes are likely to continue unless there are clear working agreements co-ordinating respective services.

Conflict over the definition of need is exacerbated by different professional ideologies. Payne (2000) highlights some of the problems of different models of intervention and the mutual distancing of health and social service staff in teams that can occur. These differences affect the way that services are delivered, as different professionals may underestimate or fail to understand the contribution of colleagues. As joint working develops, there is strong evidence that these differences may be overcome as professions work alongside one another (Smith *et al.* 1993). More problematic than professional conflicts is the development of hierarchies. Payne (2000) suggests that colleagues of different professions at similar levels in the hierarchy may have more in common than with those above or below them in their own organization. These hierarchical divisions may hinder joint working as managerial control increases over the activities of face-to-face workers. These differences in approach will not be easily handled within the proposed Care Trusts; although funding may be shared, differences are likely to emerge as to the best way to deliver services based upon medical or social models of intervention. Experience of joint working within mental health services is instructive. Shaw (2000) argues that although collaboration has a longer history in these services the medical requirement for control of patients has meant that social work has been the junior partner in working relationships so far. Given the dominance of medical models within services for older people and disabled people these may become key areas of conflict.

Conflict over priorities

Prioritizing services has led to some users being treated as problems, particularly those groups who are at risk of public stereotyping, for example, people who misuse drugs. Since their health needs have been a low priority, the NHS and the PSS have often responded inappropriately. Much community care is analysed as if it is about the major user groups. Those who require frequent, sophisticated joint service provision – for example, those with HIV/AIDS – can fall through the net as both the NHS and the PSS struggle to meet their responsibilities. The problem is greater where there are relatively small numbers of such users in a particular area. To provide a service would require greater co-ordination across authorities; this requires a central co-ordinating role. Without setting up specialist teams, local authorities do not have the expertise to meet the needs of such users, who are likely to experience even greater difficulties as they move further down the hierarchy of priorities. Some specialist teams have now been developed and it remains to be seen how effective they will be in claiming the necessary resources and co-operation to deliver more effective services.

The PSS and managerialism

As outlined above, New Labour has accepted the core arguments in favour of maintaining quasi-markets in community care. It is now striving to bring greater co-ordination to the process by developing systems of managerial control to achieve its objectives as set out in *Modernising Social Services* (DoH 1999a). This section will focus on aspects of managerial control which the present government is in the process of implementing. These are:

● performance
● standards
● quality.

Performance

There is currently a two-tier system of monitoring performance. A Best Value performance framework covering all local authority services identifies a limited set of objectives; some fifteen of them relate to the PSS, and will form part of a wider Performance Assessment Framework (PAF) covering all aspects of service delivery in the PSS.

The PAF will reflect national priorities and objectives, and therefore it is hoped that local authority performance will be measured against the performance indicators in the PAF. Local authorities will have to produce annual performance plans which should target annual improvements set against locally defined performance indicators. The Department of Health will carry out annual reviews of the social service performance plan, and the Social Services Inspectorate will carry out independent inspection and conduct joint reviews with the Audit Commission every five years (Langan 2000).

It is argued that the strength of developing performance indicators is that they provide hard figures about the performance of local authority PSS enabling performance to be measured comparatively. Thus clear evidence of improvements in practice may be gleaned from the analysis of the facts derived from the performance indicators. The problem however is in deciding on what it is you are trying to measure and whether what you have measured actually reflects improvements in performance. It is important to ask: What does the collection of such material actually measure? Allied to these more technical aspects are political concerns such as who decides on what to include as a measure and what viewpoint they adopt, for example, from the perspective of managers or users of service (Adams 1998). There are a number of problems with this approach; for example, Performance Assessment Indicator A5- emergency admission to hospital for people aged 75 and over per 1,000 of population; good performance for this indicator means keeping increases in that age group who are admitted as an emergency to hospital below 3 per cent a year:

- Will setting particular performance indicators such as reducing emergency admissions lead to activity focusing disproportionately upon crisis assessment to keep people at home while follow-up work is delayed?
- Will focusing upon assessments mean that service users with less serious needs are not dealt with, building up possible crises for the future?
- Performance indicators have to be developed in a form which can be measured and quantified; does this model fit with preventive/supportive work, i.e. work not easily measured?

- If aspects of social work practice are unable to be measured then there is the risk that it will not be a priority for employers and therefore will be of low priority or eventually disappear.

Standards

As mentioned previously, the Care Standards Act 2000 will take over responsibility for all those services regulated by local authorities (e.g. residential homes and children's homes) by creating eight regional Commissions for Care Standards. It will also take on new functions to regulate, for example:

- local authority care homes on the same basis as those in the independent sector for the first time
- domiciliary care within the mixed economy of care
- small children's homes.

In addition, the commissions will set minimum standards below which no provider will be allowed to operate. It will aim to safeguard and promote the health, welfare and quality of life of service users. This removal of the inspection function from local authorities is indicative of the way New Labour has significantly circumscribed the responsibilities of local government, given the way in which much social care will now be the responsibility of Care Trusts.

Quality

In pushing towards more managerialist approaches to quality in the PSS the assumption is that control over the product (i.e. social work services) is amenable to line management control. In making decisions about what counts as quality, managers have accrued greater power which means that issues of funding become central to the process of quality and the views of professionals and service users pushed to the margins (Lymberry 2000). This inevitably has deleterious affects upon the responsiveness to service users and communities in which they operate. As Langan (2000) argues, developing 'objective' standards of performance are largely the result of or the cause of a breakdown in community trust and the social networks which are built upon it. Thus organizations which rely on building personal relationships and co-operation between employees and service users become inhibited by the requirement to meet standards and objectives which are largely imposed from the top down. Thus as Smith (2001) has argued, the requirement to give confidence to service users by creating contracts of service in which service users have a clear idea of what levels of service to expect can undermine trust between professionals and service users. Trust requires that both parties within the social work relationship have faith in each other where a sense of uncertainty as to the outcome of service is minimized by a trust that the social worker will deliver. Contractual relationships do not have the same sense of investment in that knowing what to expect from a given level of service requires the delivery of that negotiated service; if the provider fails to deliver on contract then they are open to complaint and legal challenge. Thus performance becomes the criterion by which people are judged in relation to what they produce as defined and measurable service outcomes rather than the process of trust building and social relationships. Parton and O'Byrne (2000) draw together many studies of service satisfaction which rate process factors such as respect, being attended to and listened to as the key elements of approval from service users. Although being able to predict service outcomes and define levels of service for service users are important, social relationships between professionals and service users must also be taken into account in which relationships are built upon mutual respect and trust. Thus to ensure quality the starting point should be the evaluations of service users who may well have different measures of what constitutes service quality from those imposed by managers and central government.

Conclusion

The NHSCCA 1990 required local authorities to become enablers of community care, controlling the purchase of services and shedding their provision in social care. This changed the role and function of the PSS. They have paradoxically distanced themselves from users by divesting the provision of services to the independent sector and concentrating on the inspection and quality control of services. Social work as care management and assessment becomes a component of a wider managerial process further removed from direct user involvement. As the independent sector becomes the main provider of service, so new relationships develop with the PSS. The overlay of regulation now being instituted further centralizes control by government through divesting functions from local authorities to independent bodies such as Care Commissions which are responsible to the centre and not to local authorities. This has led some commentators (e.g. Hill 2000) to question whether the local authority PSS department has a long-term future in the light of such changes.

Key points

- Community care is contested, involving competing definitions of community.
- Community care as a product of state policy is relatively new, developing as a result of deinstitutionalization from the 1960s.
- Informal care has been a constant feature of welfare, but the explicit development of it within a mixed economy of care is new.
- Developments of the mixed economy of care involve the state as a purchaser of care, buying from private and voluntary providers.
- The role of the state as purchaser and regulator of care shifts relationships and responsibilities between the state and local authority PSS.

Guide to further reading

Sharkey, P. (2000) *The Essentials of Community Care: A Guide for Practitioners*, London, Palgrave is an accessible introduction to the subject covering the key issues. For a study in greater depth, Means, R. and Smith, R. (1998, 2nd edn) *Community Care: Policy and Practice*, London: Macmillan is the most extensive. For specific issues, Ahmad, W. and Atkins, C. (1996) *Race and Community Care*, Buckingham: Open University Press deals with a variety of concerns from an anti-racist perspective.

Chapter 6
Policy dilemmas in child and family support

OUTLINE
This chapter will:

● consider changing family patterns as they affect social work
● outline the debate between prevention and protection in child care work
● consider the refocusing of child care services
● describe specialist support for children and the implications for childcare.

The family and the Welfare State

The major political parties all regard 'the family' as central to their welfare policies and have sought in various ways to promote it. Recent concern for the family has been a response to what is considered to be its increasing fragmentation, exemplified by the rise in divorce, larger numbers of single-parent families, and non-heterosexual lifestyles. This prompted the present government to issue a consultative document upon the family, *Supporting Families* (Home Office 1998a) within which the diversity of family structure was recognized but traditional family forms given a central focus in its deliberations. More recently it has produced a magazine called *Married Life* (2001) to provide advice and guidance to newly married couples on how to maintain their marriage. In contrast to other areas of social policy, there is no recognizable department responsible for the family or any overt strategy for family life. The Labour government has continued the Conservatives' policy of maintaining parental responsibility within the family by, for example:

- encouraging single parents into work through the New Deal;
- introducing parental support orders, which reinforce parental responsibility for children who commit crime.

To explain the impact of family policy requires an analysis of the range of governmental social policies, since virtually all social policy affects the family in some way. Governments have varied in their enthusiasm for supporting the family. The aim of social policy in the nineteenth century, for example, was to enforce familial responsibility for the welfare of its members; this trend diminished following the Second World War, but has been revived since the 1980s (see Fox-Harding 1996 and Table 6.1).

Table 6.1 Changing dimensions of family responsibility

1834 Poor Law	1940 Beveridge reforms	Child Support Act 1992
Thick	Thin	Thick

Source: Fox-Harding 1996

The clearest examples of family policy may be seen within the legislation on the responsibilities of the PSS. Social workers have been intimately involved in the state's response towards the family. When the family is seen as threatened by social change, demand for social work intervention from the state increases; this occurs when: 'the assumptions that the state makes are not, or are no longer, in line with general societal perceptions of family relationships and obligations' (Fox-Harding 1996, p. 108).

From this point of view, as the family fragments, the support of children and dependent adults is threatened. Much recent legislation concerning the responsibilities of parents, in the Children Act 1989, and of carers, in the NHSCCA 1990, can be interpreted as an attempt to reinforce these responsibilities and to reduce the role of the state. These responsibilities are hardened not only through formal policy channels, but also through the creation of a moral climate, which stigmatizes alternatives to the nuclear family: 'The main problem with single motherhood is not poverty but the fact that it is an undesirable state to bring up children' (Phillips 1997, p. 104).

Where responsibilities within the family fail, or are challenged, an array of policy measures to assert the equilibrium within the family is developed. This in part involves social workers who are called upon to use their statutory powers to supervise families and sometimes remove or separate their errant members.

The return to traditional values and roles is characteristic of much modern political debate about the family. The Conservative and Labour parties have both argued for the encouragement of the nuclear family as preferable to other viable alternatives (see Home Office 1998a). Feminist writers have challenged this as underestimating the costs for women and children in maintaining often inappropriate and dangerous relationships within the nuclear family, which is now a minority family form in Britain. Despite the controversy surrounding family life, governments have relied upon the family as a major source of care (Chapter 5). They have done so both for the early upbringing of children, and in the later care of relatives with high support needs who may otherwise require state help. Support for families has usually been offered at the point of breakdown, and is often experienced as at best inadequate and at worst overtly punitive, as in the case of child protection.

Different families

Social workers are now working with different family structures, reflecting the diversity of life in this country. As Giddens (2001) suggests, families organize themselves in a variety of ways that no longer conform to a strict male breadwinner/female housewife model. Many women, for example, now live in single carer households without a male partner. The number of lone parents with dependent children has risen over the past twenty years, from 3 per cent of all families in 1971 to 7 per cent in 1998 (Giddens 2001, p. 176). To be a lone parent is to be increasingly at risk of living in poverty; some 70 per cent of female-headed, lone-parent families (90 per cent of the total) are dependent upon state support for their main income. However, these figures should be put into perspective, as the largest group who have below half average incomes, after housing costs, a generally accepted definition of living in poverty, are couples with children: some 37 per cent of the total (Kempson 1996).

These figures did not prevent the previous Conservative government from targeting single parents for attention, by attempting to recoup some of the money paid out to those on income support through the Child Support Act 1991. Invariably, single parents are women given their enforced dependent status; thus absent parents (men) were expected to financially support their former partners through a complex formula devised by the government. The complexities of the formula have been simplified to an extent by the current government and some recognition given to the diverse financial arrangements made by separated couples. However, for many critics the purpose of the Act remains: to save the Treasury money, as maintenance is taken off income support.

Social workers and social care workers have worked with the additional pressures this Act has put upon families as benefit is stopped or delayed. This has often been as a result of the overall incompetence of the Child Support Agency in calculating benefits. The Act required women to name the fathers of their children (except in circumstances which could be detrimental to the woman). This meant that some women had their benefit stopped, while others who were waiting for maintenance from their partners faced delays as this was reassessed, either through the obduracy of their partners or bureaucratic delay by the Child Support Agency. As Lewis (2001) has argued, the Child Support Agency reinforced a traditional division of responsibility by requiring the absent parent (i.e. the man) to support his children rather than to care for them.

For the PSS, differences in family organization require greater sensitivity to the different material and cultural pressures upon parents and children. For example, Pakistani and Bangladeshi people prefer to live in multi-generational households with a range of attendant concerns from wanting to maintain cultural and religious activity to a greater preference for maintaining traditional divisions of labour within families. These different family structures and cultures therefore present a range of complex challenges for social workers wishing to practise ADP. This is particularly the case for those who no longer fit traditional family structures; for example, Pakistani single-parent families find a lack of appropriate response from housing agencies, and experience lack of social support and considerable racist harassment (Beishon *et al.* 1998).

Competing perspectives and childcare policy

Different ideological perspectives have influenced policy towards children and the family. Fox-Harding (1997) lists these in the context of childcare and the PSS as:

- laissez-faire and patriarchy
- state paternalism and child protection
- modern defence of the birth family and parents' rights
- children's rights and child liberation.

Laissez-faire and patriarchy

- family is a private arena – the state should remain neutral except in extreme cases, e.g. abuse within it
- family is a haven from the outside world – relationships within it should be left alone
- adults are powerful in relation to children, men powerful in relation to women
- intervention should be minimal, and must respect the authority of parents over children unless this is clearly abused.

Current arguments

New Labour has endeavoured to bolster 'family values', favouring what it sees as traditional roles between men and women in marriage (Home Office 1998a). Ethical socialists similarly argue that crime and social breakdown are linked to absent fathers, and that the state should encourage two-parent families rather than advantaging, as they argue, single-parent families (see Dennis and Erdos 1992).

State paternalism and child protection

- The state should intervene to protect children.
- Families can damage children; the state should expect high standards of childcare.
- When parents do not fulfil their duty of care, the state must intervene.
- The interests of the child are paramount, adults' needs are secondary.

Current arguments

State paternalism was more evident in the 1960s and 1970s although it has recently been revived. Legislation currently going through Parliament (Adoption and Children's Bill) proposes quickening the pace of adoption, making it easier for adoptive parents to appeal against adverse decisions and seeks a 40 per cent increase in the number of children adopted from care.

Modern defence of the birth family and parents' rights

- The state should be proactive in supporting families through wider social policies.
- The state should provide intensive help to keep families together.
- Parental contact should continue even if a child is removed.
- Most childcare intervention is directed at working-class families.
- Most childcare problems are attributable to poverty and disadvantage.

Current arguments

Holman (1993) is closely associated with this view. Taking a strong position regarding the state and childcare, he suggests that the nuclear family should be supported by extensive state social services. These services should enable families to care for children within their own neighbourhoods. He criticizes the lack of family support by the PSS in the current climate of resource constraint.

Children's rights and child liberation

- The child's viewpoint is paramount; children have 'rights'.
- The childcare system oppresses children.
- Adults should not have power over children.
- Children are autonomous; they should be enabled to do what adults do.
- Children should not be discriminated against because of their age.

Current arguments

Of particular interest is the concern to give children in care more control over the services they receive. Children's Rights Officers are employed by many local authorities to deal with complaints from children in care and a number of voluntary groups representing children have developed childcare groups and groups to give voice to children's concerns. Paradoxically, as children's rights are beginning to be considered, more children are beginning to experience adult forms of punishment (with the lack of appropriate secure accommodation) as debates continue following the James Bulger case about the extent of children's responsibility in committing crime.

The family, child protection and the PSS

The PSS has provoked heated debate about its intervention with families, particularly those experiencing crisis. In the 1950s and 1960s, the 'problem' family was the target for social work intervention with families. As Clarke (1980) has argued, these families were seen as a residual problem, who were unable to share in the benefits of the rising material prosperity of the 1950s and 1960s. Thus a family service was to be developed so that 'they can be helped to an adjustment, and taught to catch up with the fortunate majority'

(Clarke 1980, p. 92). The focus was primarily on the problems of delinquency as a symptom of family breakdown. For example, the 1963 and 1969 Children and Young Persons Acts implied that delinquency was not something that should be dealt with by the criminal courts. Delinquency was treatable through social work with families, which was therefore more appropriate than criminalization.

Social work could address the emotional and material poverty faced by those parents unable to care for their children. This was supported by the view that the problem family was pathological, which appropriate support could restore to health. This was to be achieved by ensuring families had the material support as defined in Section 1 of the Children and Young Persons Act 1963 and in the form of casework. Social workers were to enable families to function through forms of family treatment, for example, psychiatric approaches to social work. The 'soft' intervention of counselling and therapeutic work was seen as more appropriate than strong intervention, such as the removal of children from families. There was a consensus among policy-makers and professionals alike that families were the best place for all its members. As Parton (1991, p. 20) has argued, 'the emphasis was on child care and working with the whole family'.

Parton suggests this approach was used not only with delinquency but also in early work with abused children where the goal was to nurture families to function better. The problems that emerged in the late 1970s brought these assumptions into question; these were:

- a recognition that long-term supportive work was unfocused and led to negative outcomes for children and families
- a growth in the numbers of children in care
- an increase in the use of compulsion in childcare
- wide variations across the country in practice around care decision-making
- an increase in children kept in long-term care
- a number of deaths of children, some of whom had been in care yet living at home.

(Parton 1991)

The facade of supportive and preventive work hid some disturbing elements which threw doubt on the ability of social work to normalize problem families. That social work rarely ventured into middle-class or upper-class families reinforced its residual role with working-class families.

Child abuse

Although delinquency was the major target for social work services in the 1960s, by the late 1970s problems of physical and sexual abuse dominated the agenda. The emergence of physical and sexual abuse threw doubt upon the ability of the PSS to work in a preventive way. As concern increased, child welfare services were targeted towards the detection of child abuse and the protection of children. Anxiety reached its peak in the mid-1980s, with the Parliamentary Select Committee (1984) known as the Short Report arguing that:

- the PSS had been slow to engage in effective preventive work
- there was poor quality childcare work in many social service departments
- a greater clarity between the respective rights and responsibilities of children, parents and the state was required.

It affirmed the primary responsibility of parents, arguing that the role of the state should be secondary. Parents should be given every opportunity to care for their children supported by the state, irrespective of whether the child was in care. The Report called for more prioritizing of cases, so that the small minority of families who were likely to be in danger, particularly lone-parent families, were given greater attention. This approach was confirmed by the report of the Jasmine Beckford Inquiry (1981), which recommended that 'high-risk' cases should be targeted and subject to greater intervention, including removal of children from their parents. The message at this time was for social workers to be more decisive in their actions and less ready to contemplate the rights of parents in such high-priority cases.

This approach was soon criticized by the media and politicians of all parties who felt that the PSS had become too heavy-handed in their response, specifically as a result of the Cleveland affair (see below). Support for the rights of children and parents led to the questioning of the role of the state. The rise of pressure groups championing children's and parents' rights, for example, PAIN (Parents Against Injustice) and the Children's Legal Centre, criticized the role of social workers in childcare. Intervention by professionals was increasingly placed on a par with the activities of abusive parents in the damage that could be done to the family. The view that the family is a private domain and should be supported in this by the state gained ground alongside the promotion of parents' rights.

This shift towards favouring laissez-faire and patriarchy within the family was strengthened by the Cleveland case, one of many child abuse cases that achieved notoriety in the 1980s. This case, which was highly controversial at the time, showed that parents who were alleged to have abused their children could be highly effective in mobilizing concerns about the legitimacy of child abuse work within health and social work practice. This was heightened by disagreements between the police and social services over the veracity of the claims that child abuse had taken place. The health service paediatricians and social workers involved were castigated as being over-zealous in their approach. They were accused of ignoring the rights of parents and using what the police considered to be 'unacceptable' standards of proof. Stuart Bell, Labour MP for some of the families, added fuel to the fire when he stated that the local social services had mounted an 'attack on family life'. The controversy surrounding the case resulted in the paediatricians being suspended from their posts and some of the children being returned to their parents.

Protection or prevention

Allied with the issue of rights is the question of intervention. Should family social work be about preventing general disadvantage, or should it concentrate on protecting children from abuse? The PSS has to do both; problems arise in resourcing and balancing such dual roles requiring greater breadth in intervention with families to be successful.

The state interventionist approach prevalent in the 1960s and 1970s required the PSS to prevent problems from occurring within families by providing individual and material support. Section 1 of the Children and Young Persons Act 1963 gave the PSS power to provide financial support to families if a child was in danger of being taken into care. As Tunstill (1997) argues, the optimism of the period – that social policy would promote greater welfare for all – led social workers to reduce their role in family work and provide care for children without the necessary preventive services for families.

By the 1980s, the climate of hostility towards poor families increased; responsibilities rather than the rights of parents were given prominence. In effect, this meant a targeting of reduced resources as the demands upon the PSS intensified (NALGO 1989). As more families experienced poverty, the pressures on the PSS to respond increased. The numbers of children in long-term care rose as the PSS resorted to policing families rather than using preventive methods. Such a succession of child abuse enquiries suggested that social workers had become overwhelmed by the complexity of the problems they faced. The earlier reports implied a lack of commitment to intervene, particularly where the children concerned were black, while the later reports suggested that the powers of social workers were too great, when many of the later cases involved white, middle-class families.

As ever, the local authorities and their social workers were often vilified as either neglecting problems within families which damaged children, or as over-zealous in their approach, leading to innocent families being broken up by hasty reception into care. This effectively undermined the professional status of social workers as blame swung between lack of concern or the overriding of parents' rights.

The outcome of Cleveland and other child abuse enquiries led to a tightening of guidance; for example, *Working Together* (1988) stressed:

- the need for greater inter-agency co-operation
- the need for partnership with parents to maintain family links and parental responsibility

- children should be removed when this, rather than working voluntarily with parents, advantages the child.

Childcare policy in the 1980s was subject to continual review, with different emphases being placed at different times upon the rights of children, the rights of parents, and the necessity of state intervention. For social workers it was with some relief that the government instituted a White Paper, *The Law on Child Care and Family Services* (1987), which it was hoped would deal with these issues. The Children Act 1989 that followed renewed the emphasis on parental responsibility for children.

- It required the PSS to work in partnerships with parents, keeping contact even if a child was placed into care.
- It reduced the power of the PSS to keep a child in care by extending the legal powers for parents; the period of removal of the child prior to a court hearing was reduced.

Although the Act stresses greater rights for children and parents, it does little to resolve the dilemmas between working in partnership with parents and ensuring their proper representation in court while also having to protect the rights of children. Fox-Harding (1997) argues that the balance of power has shifted towards the parents as a result of the Children Act 1989, with a recognition that the PSS should increase preventive work.

The Children Act 1989 extended the powers of the PSS to engage in the support of families outside of the care system.

- Section 17 of the Act made it a duty for the PSS to safeguard and promote the welfare of 'children in need'.
- Families should have access to supportive services of various kinds including cash payment.
- Cash assistance should take into account the ability of the family to pay back any money loaned.

The Act gave scope for other agencies, such as housing, health and education to comply with requests to help in the task of prevention if requested by the PSS, as long as this did not conflict with their statutory duties. The scope for preventive work had been widened, yet it remained unrealized.

From family support to children in need

Family support emerged in the 1980s, as a response to the implication that certain families were failing and that the PSS were failing families. The Conservative government promoted a laissez-faire concept of family which for the most part should be free from state interference, while encouraging a harsher response to families seen as failing in their duty to protect and care for their children. This message was implicit in many of the debates around the child abuse enquiries that ran in the 1980s (Clarke 1993). Although research in this period indicated the importance of a more supportive and preventive approach to families, the political climate mitigated against this. As far as the Conservative government was concerned, a more focused response was required if PSS resources were not to be stretched to unacceptable levels. This focusing upon priority families was further enhanced as a result of the Children Act 1989. Subsequent research sponsored by the Department of Health showed the process by which prioritization of resources left many families unsupported and subject to damaging and unnecessary intervention from the PSS.

Children in need

The concept of children in need (who may require a service because their health or development would be impaired without it, or who are disabled) implies, through the Children Act 1989 (Section 17), that social services departments should ascertain the extent of need of families and then prioritize their service provision. As Tunstill (1997) argues, the concept of children in need provides a filter for the previous concept of family support, and as such encourages a targeting of effort. Targeting has become more important; the majority of children on the child protection register are from families living in poverty, and those concentrated upon will be the tip of a very large iceberg of families and children living in such conditions (Figure 6.1).

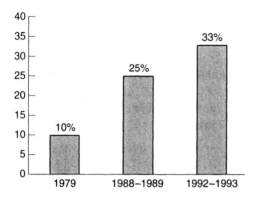

Figure 6.1 Proportion of children in population living in poverty
(below 50% average income after housing costs)

Implementing Section 17

It has been estimated that there are 600,000 children in need, of
whom about 300,000 receive some help (Dartington Social
Research Unit 1995; Little 1997). Clearly, some children in need
will not receive help; deciding who falls into this category is therefore crucial. As Dartington Research Unit (1995) has shown,
long-term emotional abuse is the most damaging environment for
children, i.e. homes that were high on criticism and low on warmth;
yet these are often the first families to be filtered out (Parton
1997b). Priority is centred on the problems of protection of children, those children considered at high risk, rather than being
children in need alone.

The demands upon the PSS have increased as governments have
recognized in principle the importance of supporting children and
families. For example, Messages from Research (Dartington Social
Research Unit 1995) showed that too much time was spent on the
investigation of child abuse, when in most cases little or no action was
taken. Too much stress was laid upon the duty to investigate under
Section 47 of the Children Act, while Section 17, which expects no
less a duty on the part of the PSS, is often seen as secondary. The
conclusion is that resources could be better used to support families,
rather than to carry out mostly futile investigations of them.

However, as Parton (1996b) argues, the encouragement of greater family support for children in need often overlooks two important factors.

1   Social work is resource limited, so families in greatest need have to take highest priority.
2   As a result of the child abuse enquiries, decision-making in childcare is based on risk avoidance.

In addressing any refocusing of children's services towards support and prevention, Parton's observations are critical. To ignore the political, legal and media pressures upon the PSS by a clarion call for refocusing is likely to repeat the failures of the 1980s. Child deaths are high profile, and politically damaging for PSS and local authorities. The recent deaths of Damilola Taylor and Anna Climbie will continue to be highly newsworthy and place social workers and their local authorities in the political limelight. This kind of attention may not encourage local authorities to spread their resources more thinly across a wider number of families. Considerable extra resourcing is required if prevention is to be effective, which in the present climate of limited resources may well require local authorities to continue to be risk averse.

Refocusing childcare

Despite the problems of resourcing and prioritization from the mid-1990s some local authorities did refocus towards more preventive responses by, for example, assessing children and families that did not involve an actual investigation for child protection. However, as noted above, this is a controversial area, and evidence to date is mixed as to the effectiveness of refocusing.

Arguments in favour

Brandon *et al.* (1999) found little difference in outcomes between cases where coercion and court action was used and similar cases where it was not. Forty-three per cent of children in the study would have been better protected without registration. English *et al.* (2000), an American study of low-risk cases, found little difference in re-referral rates between children offered an alternative service from children offered a child protection response.

Arguments against

Family support (Pringle 1998) is a generalized response compared to targeted child protection and may be inappropriate for serious cases. Parton (1996) as above criticizes refocusing as ignoring the social reality in which the public expect a more formal protectionist response. Refocusing therefore places unreal expectations upon the PSS.

Refocusing has however been reinforced by *Quality Protects* (1998) designed to enhance the management and delivery of children's services. This is a three-year programme backed by £375 million and has six priority areas for action:

1 Increasing choice of adoptive, foster and residential placements for looked-after children.
2 Improving after-care services.
3 Enhancing management systems.
4 Improving assessment, care-planning and record-keeping.
5 Strengthening quality assurance systems.
6 Consultation with young people.

A national framework for assessment of children in need is now being promoted by central government within the PSS (DoH 1999b). It is hoped that this framework will reshape practice in children's services based upon a more extensive assessment of children and families. It reflects concerns to broaden children's services response to take into account children's developmental needs, parents' capacity to respond to need, and wider social and environmental factors. Currently the assessment framework is being piloted in local authorities and will require further evaluation to assess if in the future it makes an impact upon developing a more effective response to the needs of children and their families.

In promoting more flexible and supportive responses to childcare, evidence from Europe may provide some guidance in constructing a more effective system of childcare. Baistow *et al.* (1996) show that there are fewer barriers to parents accessing support in France than at present in Britain. Hetherington *et al.* (1997) argue that procedures in this country are about filtering people out from the system, the idea of support from the PSS is seen as negative and contact with the PSS as stigmatizing. This does not apply in France and Germany, which have a more positive outlook on support from social workers (or social pedagogues, as they are called). In these countries, professionals have greater legal authority in exercising flexibility in supporting families. The result is more integration between the protection of children and family support; this provides more space in which to engage in mediation and discussion with families. This is not to say that the European experience can be transferred wholesale to Britain but it does provide alternative strategies for working on the problem of protection and prevention.

Evaluating outcomes

Gibbons (1997) suggests the following criteria for evaluating the success of the PSS in childcare:

- reduction in child deaths
- prevented harm of those children needing protection
- promotion of children's development and welfare.

Reduction in child deaths

Pritchard (1997) regards the ability to protect children from ultimate harm, i.e. death at the hand of abusers, as the main criterion. In discussing the methodological problems involved in how child death is counted and how rates have varied over time he is encouraging. He concludes that the twin approaches of prevention and protection have led to a reduction in child deaths in this country and most other industrialized countries from 1973 to the present. Pritchard's position has been contested by Gibbons (1997, p. 80), who claims that child deaths have remained 'much the same over a long period'. The discrepancy in the figures may be related to the change in how deaths were recorded; this made a considerable difference in the middle of the period under discussion. Gibbons argues that research by Creighton (1995) shows that child deaths are reduced by preventive action in reducing child mortality from accidents and infant death syndrome. It is suggested that approaches aimed at the general population may be more effective than targeted protection work with children.

Prevented harm of those children needing protection

If the reduction of child deaths is contested as a measure of success, is measuring the reduction of repeated harm of children, identified as needing protection, a more realistic goal? Gibbons argues that although studies in the UK (Dartington Social Research Unit 1995) show that between 20 and 30 per cent of children on abuse registers experienced further abuse or neglect, most involved low-level incidents with few major injuries. She concludes that it is difficult to say whether this is a measure of success or failure, as we do not know whether more children would have been injured if they had not been on the child abuse register. The difficulty is that different practices in different parts of the country reflect the different mix of services, the use of legal powers and so on, yet the outcomes remained unaffected by these differences.

Promotion of children's development and welfare

The focus upon protection noted in previous sections significantly affects the ability of the PSS to divert resources into the general support of child and family welfare. The dominance of protection is paramount in approaching children's safety, but what happens after this in terms of how children develop? As *Messages from Research* (Dartington Social Research Unit 1995) shows, social workers have been diligent in providing practical help for children but have given little attention to their developmental needs. This is particularly the case for children who are placed in care and who face considerable emotional and material disadvantages as a result (see Chapter 4).

As Gibbons (1997, p. 83) concludes, the PSS has failed to achieve any of the three outcomes: 'The evidence casts doubt on the effectiveness of current procedures in achieving any of these objectives.'

Family support and disability

The skewing of resources towards child abuse work has resulted in other areas of family support suffering. Examples are families with children who require support through a learning or physical disability, and children as 'young carers' supporting parents. Estimates as to the number of young carers vary; a recent study suggests some 30,000 children care for an adult (ONS 1997), while Barnes (1997) suggests that there may be up to 100,000 children caring for a relative.

Families with children who have disabilities have been neglected by the PSS. Despite successive attempts to encourage early involvement by the PSS in supporting such families, there has been a marked lack of positive action in this regard. The 1981 Education Act required local authorities to identify and provide a statement for children (aged between 2 and 19) who had special educational needs and to deliver an appropriate educational service for that child. This has proved inadequate since local authorities have not had the resources to meet the assessed needs of children, and have subjected parents to lengthy delays even in achieving a statement of the child's needs.

A key issue for parents and children is the transition from childhood to adulthood; at this stage in organizational terms, adults with a disability become the responsibility of the PSS. Many problems have been experienced by those transferring from education to adult social services; individuals have fallen through the net or received reduced support once they enter the adult world. This is particularly the case in day-care provision for adults, which remains underfunded relative to the resourcing in 'special' schools for children with learning disabilities. In addition, it is likely that the assessment of children's needs into adulthood often fits children into existing adult services, rather than devising opportunities for children to enter the wider adult world through, for example, work opportunities.

The 1986 Disabled Persons Act was meant to bring about a change in this situation. Sections 5 and 6 of that Act require local authorities to identify and assess the needs of disabled school leavers, but the implementation of this Act has encountered the same problems of implementation as the 1981 Education Act. As children transfer into adult services, they are typically faced by a level of provision lower than that found in the education sector. Many young adults experience increasing frustration at the inadequate levels of service operating within the adult services of the PSS.

Young carers also face hurdles, as they are often assessed as being a 'child in need' under the Children Act 1989, with their needs considered in conjunction with their parents. As Morris (1997) points out, neither parent nor child is given an assessment in their own right. This means that children and parents will not receive the specific assistance they require and to which they are entitled. The recognition that children need support in their 'caring role' of parents is central to the argument; it assumes a duty on the child to care for the parent. Yet there are significant costs associated with children caring for adults, such as:

- restricted social lives
- low educational achievement
- physical and emotional pressures of caring.

For the parent, there is the assumption that their needs can only have relevance in relation to those of the child. In effect, parents with a disability are denied the practical help they require in the home because of the focus on 'supporting' the child to be a carer. There is a danger that young carers are being inserted into the mixed economy of care in the same way as adult carers. Dearden and Becker (2000) highlight incidents of services being withdrawn from childcarers (being deemed old enough to care) leaving them without support; this echoes similar experiences of women carers. In turn, lack of support can result in children being taken into care rather than enabled to be supported with their parents in their own home.

This theme has been explored by Booth and Booth's (1994) study of parents with learning disabilities, where the issue of child support meets the rights of parents to be parents. Thus childcare workers with little experience of people with learning disabilities often intercede to 'protect' children from what they consider to be the adverse parenting of people with learning disabilities. Consistent support by the PSS is valued by parents and children in these situations, yet this is not always forthcoming, particularly where higher levels of support stretch the resource base of local social services departments. As the authors observe, it is the presence of proactive and consistent support that is the key factor in enabling parents and children to stay together. These issues are no different for parents without learning disabilities considered to be at risk, showing the importance of positive family support in enabling parents to care for their children.

Conclusion

This chapter has investigated the relationship between child protection and family support. It has argued that the focus upon the protection of children has inevitably drawn resources away from prevention and general family support. This has resulted in a refocusing of response in the UK towards more preventive strategies which seeks to redress the balance between child support and protection. It has looked at the European experience and suggested that some lessons may be learned from the experiences of countries such as France and Germany. In assessing the effectiveness of childcare and family support it has been concluded that the PSS has so far failed to meet any of the criteria for measuring effective practice in this area.

Key points

- The diversity of families requires the PSS to respond sensitively to their different forms.
- The support of families and children has increasingly been tied into child protection.
- A National Assessment Framework has been introduced which seeks to find a balance between support and protection of children.
- Support for children and families in relation to disability is given less priority in childcare.
- The recourse to guidance and procedures creates a rigidity of response which is no more successful than more flexible childcare systems in Europe.

Guide to further reading

For a general discussion of family policy, Fox-Harding, L. (1996) *Family, State and Social Policy*, London: Macmillan, is the most up-to-date. A recent training video with an accompanying reader sets out the refocusing agenda in the light of the National Assessment Framework that is well worth looking at is Department of Health (2000) *The Child's World: Assessing Children in Need*, London: Department of Health; an excellent analysis of social work in the 1980s with particular reference to the child abuse inquiries is Clarke, J. (1993) *A Crisis in Care? Challenges to Social Work*, London: Sage. Finally, a stimulating book on the differences in childcare across Europe comes from Hetherington, R., Cooper, A., Smith, P. and Wilford, G. (1997) *Protecting Children: Messages from Europe*, Lyme Regis: Russell House Publishing.

Chapter 7
Citizenship and empowerment

OUTLINE
This chapter will:

- describe universal and selective approaches to welfare
- describe the importance of citizenship for empowerment
- discuss the development of empowerment in social work
- compare competing definitions of consumerism and citizenship
- assess the importance of empowerment upon the PSS and its users.

Citizenship and social work

After the Second World War, state involvement in welfare was viewed as largely inevitable by the major political parties. The state was seen as the guarantor of the rights of individuals to a valued life. The aim was to break with the Poor Law which had blighted the operation of welfare through stigmatizing means tests and which had bitten hard in the era of mass unemployment in the 1930s (see Chapter 2). The development of universal and comprehensive social services would, it was hoped, provide social protection from the risks of living in a competitive capitalist society. The newly elected Labour government influenced by Fabian ideology wanted the Welfare State to promote citizenship and social justice for all members of society. This vision of a Welfare State excluded the PSS, which in focusing upon individual problems was seen as peripheral in determining the life chances of the majority of the population. Citizenship would be achieved by individuals claiming a universal right to, for example, social security and health care so ameliorating such social handicaps as poverty and ill health to enable maximum participation in society (see Table 7.1).

Table 7.1 Universalism

Access	Open to all
Available	To all those who have a need
Example	NHS: every person has a right to have their medical need assessed and appropriate treatment provided
Criticisms	(a) Some users gain more than others, e.g. middle classes benefit more from NHS as they have better access to services
	(b) It is argued that universal services are wasteful as some users could afford to pay for services privately

The Fabians were committed supporters of a system that would employ need, rather than a person's ability to pay as the criterion for receiving welfare. Here was a moral case to be argued as well as a practical one. The Fabians believed that selective systems required individuals to identify themselves as requiring help, resulting in a Welfare State that concerned itself only with those unable to function as individuals. This self-identification by individuals and the labelling of them by the state results in those claiming services to feel stigmatized, i.e. that their identity as persons is spoiled, resulting in feelings of shame at having to claim social benefits. To seek help is therefore a sign of failure in a society which coverts individualism and self-sufficiency. Selective systems of welfare require a complex administrative system to select those who require help which are underpinned by complex rules of entitlement. The complexity of these rules gives much discretion to officials whose job it is to make the decisions about entitlement. The complexity of selective systems coupled with the psychological and social stigmas attached to claiming prevents people from claiming what they are entitled to. However, the post-war Welfare State was still blighted by a safety net which operated upon selective principles – social assistance as it was called (now income support) became increasingly important in supplementing the incomes of the poorest as the inadequacy of universal entitlement such as unemployment benefit and the old age pension forced those entitled to such benefits to seek further help to cover their real living costs. The impact of such a selective system can be seen in the operation of income support and the social fund which results in low take-up of such benefits, as Table 7.2 shows.

Table 7.2 The stigma of seeking help

1993–1994	Range of non-take-up %	Range of those excluded 000s	Average weekly amount unclaimed £
Income support	12–21	720–1390	22.85

Source: Kempson 1976, p. 147

The acceptance of the Welfare State has been grudging in the Conservative Party; when it achieved power in 1951 antagonism simmered, but spending on welfare continued to rise (Sullivan 1996). This unease continued until the mid-1970s, when those who embraced the ideas of the New Right achieved prominence within the Conservative Party. For them altruism and voluntary effort were stifled by the heavy hand of state intervention. Personal independence and responsibility were best developed through the operation of selectivity in the Welfare State (see Table 7.3).

Table 7.3 Selectivism

Access	Only those with identified need
Available	Usually on the basis of a means test
Example	Long-term residential care: provided subject to an assessment of a person's income and savings, those with above £16,000 are responsible for all of their care
Criticisms	(a) Discourages use of services as it is based on ability to pay
	(b) Provides a minimum service for the poorest: encourages those with income to purchase maximum quality for themselves

A selective Welfare State gives no social rights to welfare; access to welfare is conditional upon the level of a person's resources, the adequacy of which is assessed by the state. Supporters of selectivity argue that this is advantageous, because it requires those above a set level of resources to make their own arrangements for welfare. It gives individuals freedom to choose what to spend their money on, unhindered by high rates of tax to pay for universal welfare. People can choose to fund their own welfare but they are not obliged to pay for others. The state will provide a minimal safety net and some help to those who, through no fault of their own, require it. Life is a risky business and individuals should not be cushioned from the consequences of their actions.

Both universalism and selectivism have been criticized as inadequate for the development of citizenship. Universalism fails to meet the different needs of a diverse population, as Langan and Ostner argue (1991, p. 139): 'treating people as though they are the same is quite different from treating them as equals.' As many feminist writers have argued (e.g. Williams 1989), the universal Welfare State gave rights in the public sphere. It was designed to ameliorate the risks to male unemployment, yet it reinforced differences of gender in expecting women to occupy the private sphere of the family. Selectivism is designed to enhance inequality between social classes based upon income. It provides a minimum of protection believing that capitalist societies increase opportunities for the majority to provide for their own welfare.

The inadequacies of universalism and selectivism have led to a sustained critique of the Welfare State. This has come from broadly-based groups such as the Women's Movement and those focused upon the use of social services such as survivors of mental health services. Within the PSS there are now a huge number of service user groups who have and continue to mount effective campaigns to give the user a voice in the organization and delivery of services. What unifies all these groups is the demand for the empowerment of service users. Empowerment is a contested subject, usually involving two opposed ideas:

1 giving greater choice for citizens, creating a consumer orientation to welfare
2 developing a voice for citizens, giving them power to decide how welfare services should meet their needs.

Over the past ten years successive governments have begun to address this issue by creating means of consultation and participation. The Citizens' Charter introduced by the previous Conservative government reflected a consumer orientation to improve access to welfare services. This has been reworked by New Labour as Service First in an attempt to place the voice of the service user at the core of service delivery by including:

- thorough provision of more detailed information on services
- transparency through service standards
- improved processes for making complaints
- regular evaluation and updating of charters.

The government is clear that its aim is one of consultation not empowerment (Powell 2001). However, in requiring local authorities to consult with service users and building this into such processes as Best Value, consultation has been given added importance in the way that local authorities manage and govern their services. The importance of citizenship in social work is in danger of being marginalized if governmental, organizational and professional preference emphasizes empowerment of service users, rather than as citizens. This is an important distinction for those who argue for a citizenship approach – if users of services are empowered within the field of social work, their rights will be limited to it. Citizens claim their rights within the political organization of society in general, and therefore their claims should not be confined to one particular social organization. In developing a citizenship approach to social work a number of dilemmas remain in pursuing such as strategy. Harris (1999) identifies these as:

- *Lack of power*. Service users of social work are often the most excluded and have little choice in using the PSS; citizenship that emphasizes choice and participation requires resources and social power which the most excluded by definition do not have.
- *Lack of market power*. In a society which values civil and political citizenship based upon individual rights and responsibilities those who lack economic power are deemed less independent

and less worthy of respect or entitlement to claim their citizenship rights.

- *Lack of status in the Welfare State.* Social work is seen as a residual service; it lacks support from the public which values mass welfare services such as NHS or state education. Thus social work is still understood as a stigmatized service for the 'unfortunate' rather than a service which everyone has a right to claim. This is reinforced by:
- *Lack of public visibility.* Social work operates between the public and the private domain in which private troubles are managed inside the family or the individual's home. Many conflicts of interest predominate, for example, between carers and cared for, whose citizenship rights often clash leaving a conflict between whose rights should prevail.
- *Lack of freedom.* Service users often have no choice about what kind of social work service they receive as they may be subject to statutory controls, for example, around childcare or mental health work. Thus they are required to comply with the power of the social workers rather than contest it as a citizen.
- *Lack of clarity and focus.* Social work covers a range of disparate and unconnected activities which militate against a clear focal point for exercising citizenship, unlike education and the school or health care and the hospital. It is thus difficult for service users to organize.

These difficulties are present in any practical application of the rights of service users within social work and provide conflicts and dilemmas for social workers and service users in their working relationships with one another. Thus in promoting citizenship social workers and service users need to understand what it is that can be achieved with empowerment through a service user approach and what can be developed with a broader conception and practice of empowerment through social citizenship.

This has been given added significance with the recognition of the importance of social exclusion, particularly in understanding the processes by which citizens become marginalized within the society in which they live. For example, Batsleer and Humphries (2000) argue that citizenship acts as a powerful exclusionary device: 'no citizenship, no entitlement, (p. 14.). The experience of many service users is therefore one in which their entitlement to services although formally in place is frustrated by barriers of exclusion such as racial discrimination, ageism and so on. For social workers committed to empowering service users, removing such barriers is crucial in linking citizenship to empowerment, enabling individuals and groups to act to achieve their definition of the good society.

What is empowerment?

CCETSW and professional bodies such as the British Association of Social Workers have enshrined ideas of empowerment and choice in their current statement of values (CCETSW 1995). Alongside these value statements is a general commitment to challenging structural oppression and discrimination. The promotion of choice and respect for individuals is the basis on which differences in power and wealth have been traditionally defended. It represents selectivist notions of welfare, in that an individual's right to choose how to dispose of their resources is given priority over notions of social justice, i.e. the equitable distribution of resources. Yet a commitment to overcoming structural oppression requires that the privileges of choice for the powerful and wealthy are secondary to the promotion of a just distribution of resources. This dichotomy reflects a serious dilemma for social workers in promoting empowerment that will be explored below.

Empowerment can be understood in two ways:

- individual
- collective.

Individual empowerment suggests that powerful professionals can relinquish power and share or transfer it to the users of services, and it has made a significant impact on community care. In focusing upon the professional relationships social workers have with users and carers, empowerment suggests ways service users can take more control of the services they require (see Table 7.4).

Table 7.4 Politics of empowerment

Individual	Collective
Confidence	Awareness of group power
Competence in social situations	Challenging social exclusion
Interpersonal skills	Collective organizational skills

These attributes are seen as worthy elements of empowerment; it is assumed that with these competences individuals will act effectively in their dealings with others and be 'empowered'. Thus social workers can employ their professional skills to enable individuals to assert themselves through group work, counselling and other interventions. The effect of empowerment can be limited if it becomes a professional technique that serves the operational requirements of social workers and their employers. Stevenson and Parsloe (1993, p. 7) explain this orientation when the term can: 'describe work with individuals and families within a relatively circumscribed context, that of their need for formal community services.'

The focus on empowerment within a service context is important and can be of considerable value for service users. Brown (1995), for example, points to the value of empowerment within the context of child sexual abuse. She argues that focusing on the criminal investigation and prosecution of offenders leaves the child victims and their carers marginalized. She suggests that work with survivors of abuse and non-abusing carers can combat the powerlessness associated with such events. Survivors are enabled to raise awareness of child sexual abuse and the right of survivors to speak out about it. This is valuable in its own right. However, proponents of the collective view of empowerment argue that individual and group approaches do not go far enough. For users to exercise power for themselves requires an overt recognition of the systematic way society oppresses them. This leads to a different understanding of empowerment as a conscious political process. It refers to a process of political action and social consciousness raising where individuals join together, as Oliver (1996, p. 147) argues, to: 'resist the oppression of others, as part of their demands to be included, and/or to articulate their own views of the world.'

Collective empowerment is a process of winning power; it is not something given by those in authority. The goal of empowerment is to work for the inclusion of marginalized groups as fully participating citizens. Some disabled people's organizations, for example, have campaigned for wide-ranging anti-discriminatory legislation to prevent society from denying opportunities for the social inclusion of disabled people (Oliver and Barnes 1998). Similarly, Survivors Speak Out has challenged the way mental health services have adopted gendered, ethnocentric and medicalized views of mental health which have reflected and led to society-wide devaluing of people with mental health problems.

Consumers and citizens

In building empowering practices, organizations have developed different ways of relating to their service users. The PSS are being influenced by the reorganization of local government particularly in the requirement to consult with service users which requires them to develop new systems of accountability to the population they serve. For the previous Conservative government this meant service users becoming consumers of privatized services to exercise choice through their purchasing power. As a result, service users now have a different relationship with the PSS, with the implication in theory that they have the power to choose which kinds of service meet their individual needs from a range of alternative service providers (see Chapter 5). The theory assumes that individual consumers will be able to change from one provider to the next, exercising their power of 'exit'.

This model may be compared to a citizen-based approach. The latter suggests that users of services should have more say or 'voice' in the development and delivery of services. This means in theory more input at every stage of their production and consumption, thus requiring high levels of commitment from service users towards consultation and participation within the organizational structures of PSS (see Figure 7.1).

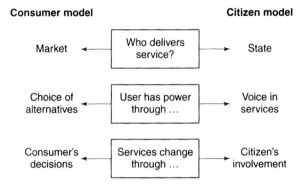

Figure 7.1 Models of empowerment: consumers and citizens

Problems of consumer and citizen models

The competing models highlight a number of practical concerns. The consumer model begs the following questions:

- Are the consumers of public services similar to those in private markets?
- Can consumers of public services make similar choices to those in private markets?
- Are the constraints on consumers' choices of public services subject to different constraints from those in private markets?

The problems of a consumer approach

There are differences for consumers of social work services; first, they do not always have a choice as to whether they receive a service. Social work has a statutory duty to intervene where children or adults are at risk in some way. The parents of a child suspected of child abuse do not have the right of exit in determining whether they want the service of a social worker. The nature of the public task, i.e. protection of vulnerable individuals and the control of damaging environments, removes the idea of choice. Those not subject to statutory services face other hurdles. To make effective choices, knowledge of alternatives to exit service provision is essential; for many this information is not readily available. They are often in a vulnerable position, requiring a particular service quickly; if it is not forthcoming, it is likely to cause great discomfort. Possible solutions to these dilemmas have developed around the idea of quasi-markets, which in theory do not have the same characteristics as private markets, as Table 7.5 shows.

Table 7.5 A comparison of private and quasi-markets as service provision solutions

Private markets	Quasi-markets
Buyers' competition	Monopoly competition
Sellers' competition	

Quasi-markets differ from private markets in the role of the buyer/purchaser of service, which is taken by the public authority and not the individual consumer. In social work this is developed through the purchase of contracts of service from private/voluntary providers supervised by a care manager. It is the care manager who is the purchaser of the service and the user who consumes it. This requires the user to have some power other than through exit, as he/she does not have an initial choice over which service to purchase.

Consumers of public services in quasi-markets are therefore subject to different constraints from those in private markets. Consumers of the PSS are not always able to make an informed choice between alternative services. An older person who is at crisis point, needing services to remain in their own home, may not have the facility or the physical capacity to shop around for appropriate services. The consequences for purchasers are potentially severe. Consumers purchasing inappropriate residential care, for example, can experience loss of freedom, poor physical and psychological health, and neglect by staff leading to physical abuse or worse.

The problems of a citizen approach

The effectiveness of the citizenship model has also been questioned.

- What influence will a person have over how services are planned?
- How much say will a person have over the way services are delivered?
- How will groups of service users express their voice in service delivery?
- How are groups of service users to acquire a voice in the planning of services?
- Do different users have different requirements of empowerment?

Service users are encouraged to be involved through the care management process in participating in their own care plans. The NHSCCA 1990 argued that services would be developed around the needs of individuals rather than individuals being fitted into existing services. For this, the user must be included as a partner in the assessment process. This has been problematic (see Chapter 5); local authorities have prioritized services and rationed assessment and provision. Once assessment has taken place the experience has not, in general, been one of partnership or empowerment. Ellis (1993) researched users' understanding of assessment and showed that their experience was a negative one. They were confused by the process, and voiced their cynicism about the purposes of the PSS in involving them in what they perceived as a tokenistic exercise.

The extent to which users control service delivery is problematic. For users who wish to change services, or the time at which they are provided, local authorities remain inflexible. Local authorities increasingly provide only core services; those requests that do not fit into existing provision are left to the private sector, which provides, for example, social care at the weekend or in the evening. More flexible services, such as the now-defunct Independent Living Fund, proved popular because those who received it could organize their own care arrangements, by buying their own care at the times they wanted. Greater flexibility can be achieved if local authorities take advantage of the Direct Payments Act (1996), though as Pearson

(2000) has argued the schemes she studied were still subject to much control and inflexibility of management, for example, by restrictive rules as to how money could be spent on direct care. Policy guidance following the NHSCCA 1990 required local authorities to consult not only other agencies involved in delivering services but also carers' and users' groups. Local authorities have been slow in responding to this guidance: few have involved users and carers at the planning stage in developing community care plans.

In enabling users to exercise their voice, local authorities will have to open up the process of planning service provision. This requires more time and resources to be placed into negotiating and finding out from users what they want. This means attending to the process of empowerment rather than, as Barnes (1997) has argued, the production of a planning document. Crucial to this approach is deciding who will be consulted. There are the traditional representatives of users with long-standing relationships with local authorities, for example, Age Concern and MENCAP. But what of newer organizations consisting of users themselves who are demanding a greater voice in the planning process?

Effective planning is an ongoing process. Users and carers are expected to maintain what can be a demanding schedule of meetings, while balancing their other responsibilities. This means, for example, maintaining a valued lifestyle alongside their commitment to user empowerment. It may also divert valuable time away from wider campaigning and raising issues in society. Relatively few users will have the resources to maintain such a commitment without the active support of the local authority to sustain them. Essential to this commitment is that local authorities take the contribution of users seriously, so that recommendations or issues raised by them are not lost in the planning process.

In enabling users to develop a voice, there are problems if users are seen as an undifferentiated group. Users have different interests that are not always reconcilable with one another; the needs of carers and users may not always match; carers and users may want conflicting outcomes from the process of consultation. For example, Rescare campaigns on behalf of some carers of people with learning disabilities to develop specialist residential facilities, such as village communities, which they see as valued resources. Against this, organizations such as People First and Values into Action argue for the opposite – the further integration of people with learning disabilities into the community.

Similarly, the particular needs of different user groups should be recognized; people with learning disabilities or physically frail older people will have different needs from survivors of mental health services, or people with disabilities. For example, those with greater skills in and opportunities for communicating can dominate any consultation process. This is clearly an issue between many isolated, frail, older people and more mobile and less isolated users. Carers in this regard have been able to dominate consultation processes at the expense of users.

In concentrating upon the public face of empowerment there is a danger of overlooking the private aspects of such a process. Barnes (1997) argues that there are many ways in which users take on valued and empowering roles within their everyday lives such as carer, parent or lover that can often be ignored in the focus upon formal consultation over services. Just as feminist writers have argued (see Chapter 3) for the importance of valuing women's contribution within the private sphere of the family, so users in their everyday lives need similar recognition. For example, parents with disabilities require the same valued opportunities to parent their children as anyone else and to be seen as having needs in their own right. This means, as Morris (1997) argues, that parents with a disability should be assessed in terms of their needs as an individual and a parent. Often their children's needs are assessed as a young carer and therefore a 'child in need' under the Children Act 1989. This raises serious questions about the needs of disabled persons to be parents and carers for their children rather than vice versa. It also raises issues about the rights of children not to be required to take on demanding caring roles which may impact upon their education attainment and social relationships; for example, becoming socially isolated through their caring duties.

Community care and empowerment

Best Value (Department of the Environment 1998) requires local authorities to develop procedures for consulting users in all their services. Since the early 1990s local authorities, as a result of the 1990 NHSCCA and now Best Value, have slowly developed strategies for what they consider to be participation and consultation of users, but as noted above this does not mean empowerment. A commitment to empowerment requires local authorities to open up their own organizations to change and involve service users at every level of the organization. Local authorities need to provide information, help users attend meetings and be clear what areas of decision-making are open for consultation. PSS need to support users and their own staff, give time to the process of consultation and commit all levels of their organization to respond positively to the decisions users wish to enact.

Initiatives to develop empowering practice by local authorities are to be welcomed; there is evidence that local authorities are developing such approaches (Barnes 1997). However, there is still much to be accomplished in developing relationships between users, professionals and the organizations involved. Servian (1996) suggests that for service organization and delivery to be focused upon service users the following should be present:

- perceived control by participants
- perceived positive encouragement of users and carers
- perceived positive value of the individual and of the social group of which the individual is a member
- encouraging users to speak out which is valued by managers and professionals
- real and open access to choice
- meetings to operate on the basis of open agendas, plain language and shared/equal membership
- power structures to be transparent: hierarchies and decisions to be made at all levels should be open to view and challenge.

For some user groups the problem they face in finding a voice within the PSS may be overcome through a different approach to empowerment. This requires that the users themselves have the power to decide on their own services through the provision of direct payments so that they can buy services to meet their preferred needs. This approach has been promoted by disabled people who see within it the opportunity to gain their independence from what they consider to be the disablist practice of the PSS. The Disabled Persons Act 1986 gave disabled people a right to an assessment of their needs for practical assistance in the home, along with aids and adaptations to enable daily living. This assistance was covered by the Chronically Sick and Disabled Persons Act 1970, but was not adequately implemented by most local authorities.

However, some local authorities, such as Sheffield, began to provide direct payments to users on an experimental basis. This was particularly successful, and under continued pressure from disability groups, the Conservative government introduced the Independent Living Fund in 1988. This was intended to be directed at a small number of disabled people who had been affected adversely by changes to Income Support as a result of the Social Security Act 1986. However, with the popularity of this provision, the numbers using the fund (and therefore expenditure on it) rose until it was stopped for new claimants in 1993, when it had reached 21,500 people who received a total of £100 million. With its popularity proved, the government suggested that it would look into ways of providing this facility through local authorities; again after much pressure from various welfare groups, a new scheme was approved.

What followed was the Direct Payments Act 1996 that empowered local authorities to set up direct payment schemes. However, the scheme is hedged with qualifications as to how the direct payments may be made. The implications of opening up the potential demand from users led local authorities to be very cautious in their approach. Initially, the scheme is to be restricted to those with physical impairments and learning disabilities. The provisions of the Act keep the power of decision firmly in the hands of the local authority by enabling local authorities to:

- means test users, so offsetting the potential cost on to the individual
- decide who is willing and able to use the service
- require agreement from the user on how the money will be spent

- require that the bought-in service cannot be provided or arranged cheaper by the local authority
- allocate funding according to the level of disability.

This gives a high level of control to local authorities through the assessment, monitoring and gatekeeping of direct payments (Pearson 2000). Thus the PSS can continue to manage the process through such gatekeeping functions as limiting the amount of control disabled people would require from direct payments. Those from a disability rights perspective emphasize the increased choice and flexibility that direct payments bring (e.g. Morris 1997), while others (e.g. Ungerson 1997) suggest that direct payments are not a panacea, emphasizing the potential exploitation of carers (see Table 7.6).

Table 7.6 The debate over direct payments

In favour	*Against*
● Empowers disabled people	● Disempowers carers as casual workers
● Gives choice/flexibility	● Encourages poorly trained carers
● Reduces dependency on PSS	● May encourage exploitative/ oppressive relationships
● 30%–40% cheaper than equivalent provided services	● Encourages low-waged care work

The Direct Payments Act 1996 confirms the general trend of the PSS withdrawing from the direct provision of services and moving towards an enabling role. What is interesting about this is that the mixed economy becomes further complicated as users take their place within it as employers of services for themselves alongside the independent sector. This is potentially empowering for service users, yet it may also raise additional questions about the employment of carers within a labour market that has traditionally been a highly exploitative one, particularly for women.

Enabling and empowerment

The development of the enabling role of the PSS, in which they are responsible for the co-ordination of a mixed economy of care, poses new challenges for social workers. Empowerment of service users in the provision of service becomes problematic when the PSS themselves no longer provide the bulk of services. Managers in the PSS and social workers are developing new methods of working with providers in the voluntary and private sectors. Although the NHSCCA 1990 encouraged local authorities to consult users, they are rapidly losing the bulk of their services to the independent sector. This makes the realization of empowerment uncertain.

- How are local authorities to empower users of services which, for the most part, they do not provide themselves?
- Can they use their power within the contracting process to ensure that consultation is carried out by the providers they contract with?
- Do they keep consultation only at the planning stage?

Part of the answer could be in the development of partnerships with user groups. The Derbyshire Centre for Integrated Living (DCIL) (managed by the Derbyshire Coalition of Disabled People and the local authority) enables disabled people to buy in services contracted from the Centre. This places the resource under the joint control of the local authority and the Coalition while ensuring that there is a collective interest in the nature and quality of services. This resource opens up opportunities for people with disabilities, since the Centre itself defines the kinds of service that are appropriate, in partnership with service users who have a voice in the organization of the resource. This is clearly different from voluntary providers which work and speak on behalf of people with disabilities, but do not necessarily involve disabled people themselves. Priestley (1998) in his study of self-assessment processes within the DCIL shows the potential for challenging narrow professional assessments based upon assumptions of the dependency of disabled people to one of self-empowerment where disabled people participate in managing their own affairs.

Assessment and empowerment

The difficulties experienced by users involved in need assessments are at the heart of the debate regarding empowerment. The direct contact of the PSS with users in negotiating the level of need and service to be provided is at issue here. Social workers' ability to work in an empowering way through the assessment process is becoming harder and depends upon:

- the pressures from their managers to be circumspect in their needs assessments
- the difficulties they face in working collaboratively.

While expecting to be able to empower users, social workers are required to carry out their duties of assessment in a culture of resource constraint. Reduced budgets require greater rationing of services, which can leave departments open to legal challenge if the assessments that are carried out fall short in the provision of service. The rise of legal challenges to local authorities is an example of a lack of empowerment of service users, if users need recourse to lengthy and expensive legal challenges to contest decisions made by the PSS. The House of Lords, ruling in favour of Gloucester Social Services Department in 1997, is one example. Age Concern challenged the way the local authority reduced services without any reassessment of users' needs. The ruling allowed Gloucester to take into account their overall level of resources in deciding to:

- make an initial assessment of a service user's need
- to reassess a service user's need.

Challenges from the courts are likely to continue as resources remain scarce. This is likely to limit areas of discretion, so that local authorities will deliver rationed services to priority users based on tighter, but more transparent, criteria to avoid legal challenge. *Modernising Social Services* (DoH 1999a) mirrors these issues by requiring a national charging system which it argues should be equitable and transparent. However, as Stanley (1999) argues, the voice of service users who have higher needs is often lost in the process of assessment which limits discretion of social workers through restrictive assessment forms, lack of service resource and sheer volume of work. This leaves only the most articulate, vocal and active service users to have their needs considered but not necessarily met.

The limiting of social workers' ability to work in more empowering ways has been felt particularly within childcare through the rationing of social work in child protection. Approaches to empowerment within childcare have consistently faced the problem of reconciling the duty to protect children with the duty to provide supportive and preventive services. In childcare, social workers find it increasingly difficult to work in a collaborative way with users, especially since the Children Act 1989 and the support for 'children in need' (see Chapter 5).

Jordan (1997) suggests that there are clear problems in developing more empowering practice with families and drawing them into partnership with statutory social work. As social workers have been channelled into protection work, the space to work with users in more empowering ways is lost; as a result a greater distance develops as:

- much family support is delivered by family support staff with fewer qualifications
- support is increasingly delivered within voluntary organizations.

Parents who were interviewed by Jordan (1997) in a family centre recognized this distinction, in which child protection work was seen as unconnected to family support work. The staff whom Jordan studied were either seen by parents as friendly and supportive (involved in family support work), or formal and exclusive (and therefore child protection workers). The wider implications for empowerment are profound. Jordan argues that trust and collaboration will falter if the childcare service is split between family support and child protection. Parents will continue to view those workers in child protection with suspicion, as they will always be dealing with controlling aspects of childcare. Thus an occupational and organizational distance has developed between what should be parts of the same service to children. Protection work is organized within statutory social services, while family support is increasingly placed within the independent sector. Statutory work largely becomes the province of trained social workers. Family support is managed by a core of professionally trained workers with an array of untrained and/or voluntary workers providing face-to-face support. This has led to guidance being issued by successive governments to attempt to re-focus the work of statutory services towards a more supportive orientation, as early in 1994 government bodies were urging local authorities to promote a wider range of initiatives to provide families with more social support (Audit Commission 1994). Government sponsored research echoes these views and has called for a reconsideration of the way in which professionals are perceived by parents who are accused of abusing or neglecting their offspring, thus giving parents more sense of control over their involvement and the services they received (see Parton 1997b)

Evaluating empowerment

From the evidence presented, we have outlined a number of problems with empowerment. The initiative has flowed from the PSS to involve users in a process that is controlled to a large extent by them and not the users. There is a danger that empowerment becomes an expression of the PSS's power over users. This is a paradox, as Baistow (1995) suggests, in that users become the objects of empowerment: it is something done to them, rather than becoming subjects so that they themselves can take control. For example, developing parenting programmes for 'inadequate' parents, or controlling what might be considered inappropriate behaviours of people with learning disabilities through group work is not empowerment. These initiatives may be legitimate depending on the circumstances, but they cannot be interpreted as empowering users of service; rather the opposite in that they are about controlling behaviour which is considered unacceptable or inappropriate. Clark (1998) in his study of social workers' attitudes to empowerment reinforces the argument, observing that stronger collective approaches to empowerment have little currency at present with social workers who continue to have a limited conception of consultation and an individualistic understanding of client need.

As Croft and Beresford (1997) argue, users' involvement has been steered to planning and management issues, whereby they are drawn into the bureaucratic structures of PSS departments. Thus the opportunity to consider social work practice itself and its effects upon users is lost. As they suggest, empowerment is experienced as 'stressful, diversionary and unproductive' (Croft and Beresford 1997, p. 275); it can result in further alienation of users rather than inspiring them to take more control for themselves. For professionals to develop empowering forms of practice requires a commitment from themselves and their employers to develop practice and procedures that involve users and change the culture of their organizations. This means that empowerment becomes an everyday, commonplace and integral aspect of what social workers do. It is both integral to social work practice in which the user's voice is valued and their story given validity (Parton and O'Byrne 2000), and part of the wider goals and objectives of the organization and society at large. Empowering users is not something that should be within the control of the PSS alone, it should be user led. As user groups themselves suggest, the position of disempowered people will not be solved through appropriate social work or social care alone. It requires a process of civil rights in which the disempowered take their place in society as citizens who take power for themselves.

Conclusion

This chapter has placed empowerment within a wider societal context. It has discussed two competing conceptions of empowerment within the PSS which are contested notions of citizenship. It has analysed the difficulties in empowering the users of the PSS and discussed how both the exit and voice models have their own unique problems. Finally, it has assessed the effectiveness of empowerment and the increasingly politicized nature of this concept for the PSS and the users of service.

Key points

- Empowerment within the PSS is based upon two competing models: exit and voice.
- Empowerment is a wide-ranging concept involving the sharing, transfer and taking of power between professionals, the state and user groups.

- Empowerment may be characterized as individual or collective.
- PSS need to develop empowerment as part of their strategic thinking.
- For empowerment to be effective it must be an expression of social citizenship.

Guide to further reading

In discussing the implications of citizenship, social policy and social work Powell, F. (2001) *The Politics of Social Work*, London: Sage, provides a well-written account of the issues. For a discussion in relation to theories of empowerment and the PSS, Servian, S. (1996) *Theorising Empowerment: Individual Power and Community Care*, Bristol: Policy Press, is an excellent introduction. For a view of users' concerns Beresford, P. and Turner, M. (1997) *It's Our Welfare: Report of the Citizens' Commission on the Future of the Welfare State*, London: NISW, provides a challenging account.

Chapter 8

Social work in altered circumstances

OUTLINE
This chapter will:

● analyse support for the PSS and the Welfare State
● assess the record of the former Conservative government in respect of the PSS
● explore New Labour's approach to the Welfare State
● assess New Labour's social policy for the PSS.

Social work and the Welfare State

All the main political parties assert that the Welfare State must change to respond to the challenges of the global economy. They argue that the sweep of technological, social and economic development has challenged previous orthodoxies, particularly the role of the state in delivering welfare. Social work, like other Welfare State services, has changed as government has responded to these demands. Previous chapters have highlighted some of these demands, including:

● an excluded minority of the population (some 30 per cent) reliant upon state benefits;
● an increasing proportion of the population aged 75 and over;
● changes in family structures increasing the proportion of single carer households;
● increasing desire for culturally appropriate welfare services;
● the dominance of market solutions to the problem of welfare.

In response, social work now operates within a different set of social and political assumptions from that of thirty years ago, as Table 8.1 shows.

Table 8.1 The changing nature of social work

	Post-Seebohm	Post-2000
Social work process	Social work is skilled helping	Social work is managing practical help
	Social work is universalist	Social work is selective
	Social work is client-centred	Social work is consumer-oriented
Social work organization	Integrated social service departments	Mixed economy of care
	Main providers	Change to purchasers
	Regulate own services	Inspects/regulates mixed economy
Organizing principles	Mass provision	Individualized care packages
	Institution-based services	Community-based services
	Within local authority	Within local mixed economy
	General support for citizenship	Consumer empowerment
Role of welfare	Provision of public welfare service	Enabling a mixed economy of care
	Develop rights to community service	Develops responsibilities to self/family and community
Service delivery	The state	Markets and quasi-markets
	Family as supplement	Family central to service provision
	Voluntary/private sector (minimized)	Voluntary/private sector (maximized)

Recent policy in the PSS has reduced expenditure relative to demand, and developed alternative approaches to service delivery through reducing the state provision of services and expanding the independent sector. This has reduced and redirected state activity through:

- the containment of spending
- privatization
- quasi-markets
- centralization.

The containment of spending

Government pressure on local authorities to reduce spending has cut the provision of the PSS. While in real terms spending on the PSS has grown by 48 per cent, from £3.6 billion in 1990 to 1991 to £6.4 billion in 1994 to 1995, demand has increased, as have the costs of delivering services (Bebbington and Kelly 1995). Much of the increase in funding has involved the transfer of money to local authorities to meet their community care responsibilities. Public information is inadequate in this respect, but there have been some attempts to estimate the extent of underfunding. George (1996) showed, for example, that the money passed to local authorities by central government through their Standard Spending Assessments (SSAs) was on average 6 per cent lower than in 1994 to 1995, while over the period 1993 to 1996, SSAs declined by nearly 5 per cent. The Conservative government's strategy was to contain expenditure in the belief that there were significant gains to be made in efficiency savings. Reducing expenditure forces local authorities to find new ways of making fewer resources go further. After a sustained period of cost containment, it is unlikely that significant gains can be made without damaging service provision. For example, by 1997 local authorities were spending on average 7 per cent more on community care than the SSA set by central government, within a culture of strong rationing of resources and prioritization to high-risk cases. This pressure leads local authorities to find alternative ways of meeting need outside their own provision.

Since the election of New Labour there has been some increase in overall expenditure; spending had increased from £7,324 million in 1995/1996 to £8,940 million by 1998/1999, representing a 2 per cent increase as a total of local authority spending. This increase has been fuelled in part by the government providing specific grants to modernize the PSS as part of *Modernising Social*

Services (DoH 1999a), for example, providing some £75 million for children's services.

Local authority budgets are tight when the increased demand and expectations of its services are taken into account. New Labour appears to be targeting money for specific purposes into the PSS and from which local authorities are required to spend this extra money in prescribed ways as part of the modernizing agenda. This has led many local authorities to spend over budget as they struggle to meet the government's priorities; this has been particularly severe in children's services where the impact of Quality Protects has resulted in significant spending problems (Community Care, 1 February 2001). Taking public expenditure in total, New Labour has been an enthusiastic guardian of the public purse. It adopted the Conservative expenditure plans in the first two years of office and will continue to keep spending under tight control; thus in 1991/1992 total spending by government was 42.2 per cent of GDP, and even by 2003/4 public spending will be only 40.6 per cent. Investment in the Welfare State has also been subject to firm control and has increasingly involved public–private partnerships (PPP) in which private consortia provide capital for current investment in building and services, in return for future repayments on their capital outlay. For example, hospital building for the NHS will result in future payments by the state to the private sector, thus the state will be paying some £3.5 billion a year from 2004/2005 to 2012/2013 to private consortia to finance ongoing investment in hospital building (Toynbee and Walker 2001). This represents a dearer way of investing in public services in the long term than if the state borrowed the money from financial institutions in the first place. As part of some PPPs it has also involved the running of support services to be placed over long-term contracts to further finance the deals, leading to long-term control of public services (twenty-five to thirty years) being placed into the hands of private contractors with minimal safeguards (Monbiot 2000). Research by Ball *et al.* (2001) confirms the problems with this approach to financing investment in the Welfare State, suggesting that any initial gains in the short term are likely to be lost.

Privatization

The 1980s saw significant funds from the social security budget move into the subsidizing of private residential care. This expansion is problematic for local authorities and the private sector, largely as a result of the NHSCCA 1990 which:

- controlled access to private care through local authorities assessing all those requiring financial help
- compelled local authorities to spend 85 per cent of the transferred budget in the private or voluntary sector
- developed a mixed economy of care, whereby the monopoly purchaser – the local authority – contracts with private and voluntary providers for services.

Within the new managed quasi-markets the expansion of private care has slowed and the profits in this sector have declined. As local authorities cut back on their service provision and tendering for services to the private sector, so the service base in the mixed economy erodes.

One of the major effects of privatization has been upon the social care workforce. Savings derived from developing privatization were to come from the 'expensive' wages and conditions of service in the local authority sector. These savings may be harder to achieve. As the Labour government maintains its policy of a minimum wage, both private proprietors and some local authorities fear the impact of increased wage costs on their contracts. Other local authorities have welcomed the minimum wage, seeing it as levelling the playing field, so that local authority services will be able to compete when wage costs between the private and local authority sector are taken into account. As Hirst (1997b) points out, this poses a moral dilemma; low wages discourage committed or appropriate staff from applying for work in social care, yet the impact upon local authorities already starved of cash increases the amount spent on the private sector for care services.

Privatization is now an important feature within the domiciliary and day-care sector (see Chapter 6). Local authorities are prioritizing their services, encouraging those whose needs are seen as less pressing to pay for private domiciliary care or charging for their own care services. George's (1996) survey shows the number of community care assessments where those assessed who received a service fell by one-third, from 6 per cent to 4 per cent between 1993 to 1994 and 1996 to 1997. This was confirmed by social service directors, who felt that the eligibility criteria for getting a service had toughened over the past three years. Likewise, the Audit Commission's (2000) report on charging shows the extent of self-provision through charging service users, so that 94 per cent of councils, for example, now charge for home care services.

New Labour has no strong ideological commitment to the public sector within local authorities. What is important are outcomes; thus the delivery of the service and the processes involved can take place in the independent or the local authority sector. The expectation that local authorities should continue to prioritize efficiency, economy and effectiveness is used not necessarily to remove services into the private sector but is intended to act as a spur to local authority provision to match what is considered to be the best level of service within the independent sector. New Labour continues to search for more opportunities to privatize parts of the Welfare State; their manifesto *Ambitions for Britain* (Labour Party 2001) for the 2001 election outlined proposals to privatize many of the administrative services of the NHS, public–private partnerships to develop treatment centres, and more private/public partnerships are suggested for the delivery of education and social care.

Quasi-markets

Privatizing the residential care market in the 1980s led to the creation of 'perverse incentives'; individuals who could have remained at home were subsidized to enter private care via the social security system. The introduction of a quasi-market into community care was intended to provide the necessary control through the PSS assessing and monitoring the mixed economy within a social care market. The Joint Reviews of Local Authorities (1997), however, criticized local authorities for not achieving a balance between ensuring a supply of appropriate social care services and encouraging competition between providers. This has resulted in high transaction costs for local authorities and a greater unreliability for users. The supply of such services is subject to greater volatility, as some local authorities switch between providers to cut costs.

The effect of quasi-markets is also beginning to be felt within children's services, as local authorities move towards a core child protection service while purchasing services for residential and family support from the independent sector. Petrie and Wilson (1999) have charted the way children's services are being drawn into a market framework with virtually all children's day care now provided by the independent sector and some 50 per cent of fostering services now placed within a purchaser/provider framework. The development of private fostering agencies is a significant challenge to local authorities as private agencies are able to provide better support and remuneration for their foster carers. The result has been foster carers moving from the local authority to private agencies which are then offering packages of foster care back to local authorities.

Centralization

Paradoxically, the 1980s saw the greatest centralization of power to the state since the Second World War, given the anti-state ideology of successive Conservative governments in the 1980s (Jenkins 1995). As Taylor-Gooby (1996) argues, central government has traditionally set the broad framework for the Welfare State, while the planning, delivery and day-to-day management was the responsibility of local authorities. Social work professionals had a high degree of autonomy within the local authority structure relative to other areas of local government. What had emerged by the 1990s was a process of 'nationalization' of power, with control shifting further towards central government (Jenkins 1995). Removing the power of local authorities to levy taxes independently through the rates was crucial. Local authorities became dependent upon central government's assessment of their needs, and this has seen local authorities penalized for overspending by losing grants the following year.

Centralization has also been achieved by changes in local government administration. The breakup of the large metropolitan authorities such as the Greater London Council in the mid-1980s has been carried forward into local government generally with the development of unitary bodies based upon smaller geographical areas of administration. Some observers believe these smaller authorities will be able to co-ordinate the activities of different welfare services as they will overlap within the unitary body, for example, between health, housing and social services. Others argue that the further fragmentation of administration will make it harder to co-ordinate different arms of PSS activity, particularly in child protection. The prospect of smaller populations means that it will be harder to generate the necessary local income to run the services required. In addition, the political strength of local authorities will be weakened as they represent a smaller local electorate, so reducing their bargaining strength with the centre (Adams 1996). It is unclear at present whether the proposed regional governments will be able to, for example, reorganize the provision of local authorities to make co-ordination of services more effective or indeed whether they will have greater powers placed with them than currently pertains to local authorities.

To cut back on funding and reorganize the way the PSS is delivered within quasi-markets is one way to maintain central control. However, as noted in previous chapters on child and community care, central government has sought additional control of the activities of local authorities and the social workers employed by them. It has done this by:

- increasing the prominence given to inspection and quality control through, for example, the SSI
- publishing performance measures
- the proliferation of guidelines and procedures to ensure compliance to notions of best practice
- expanding the activities of the Audit Commission.

This process is complex – arms-length inspection via the SSI and investigation by the Audit Commission combine with new managerial processes of quality control and performance measurement to develop new forms of governance over the PSS. To the extent that the state exercises arms-length control via these agencies, overall strategic command is kept centrally, with an increasing role for bodies such as the SSI in overseeing the operational side of the PSS.

New Labour has supplemented this process by removing more functions from local authority PSS departments. In creating such bodies as Regional Care Commissions to monitor and inspect care standards and giving more control of social care to the NHS through the setting up of Care Trusts, New Labour appears to have as much scepticism towards the ability of local authorities to manage services effectively as did the Conservatives. By doing so they have augmented the centralizing tendencies under the previous government; as Jordan and Jordan (2000) have argued the difference is that under the Conservatives these centralizing tendencies were moderated by the power of the market and individual consumer choice to limit the power of bureaucrats and professionals. Under New Labour's regime the power of the centre is augmented by the resort to strong regulatory structures such as performance assessment frameworks, to require compliance by local authorities with the policy goals of the centre.

New Labour and the Welfare State

The Labour Party has responded to these new conditions by reinventing itself as New Labour, and creating a significant distance from the state-oriented approach of Fabianism. New Labour has outlined a strategy for the Welfare State which uses social policy to develop social investment in order to expand growth within the economy. New Labour accepts that within a globalized world economy governments have less control over their own economic development than they had previously. National governments must compete to attract inward investment from multinational corporations with a range of benefits such as government grants and subsidies to enable a 'favourable business climate'. Thus the old manufacturing industries find difficulty in surviving when corporations can close down their operations in one country to reinvest in developing areas where there are large pools of labour which are more exploitable, costing significantly less in wages, conditions of work and social benefits. These countries' workers lack the protection of such organizations as trade unions to fight for decent pay and working conditions, and combined with high levels of absolute poverty, people are desperate for work. Multinational companies can capitalize upon the opportunities that globalization brings to increase profits and dividends to their shareholders.

The impact of globalization upon social work and social care has generated much debate and has revolved around those who argue that globalization is a strong force influencing the shape of the PSS in its organization and service delivery as against those who suggest that globalization is not the all-encompassing force that its proponents suggest. Khan and Dominelli (2000) argue for a strong association between the forces of globalization and its impact upon social work. Thus many of the changes outlined in previous chapters of this book in relation to adult and children's services may be linked to the pressures of globalization. For example, the continuing privatization of social care is attributed to the pressures on national governments to keep their social costs low to create fewer demands for taxation upon multinational companies considering investing in the UK. The increased regulation and control from central government is likewise seen as significant in creating more responsive forms of organization that can encourage greater effectiveness and efficiency in service delivery, expressed through policy such as Best Value. Contrary to this argument, Pugh and Gould (2000) suggest that the acceptance of changes to the Welfare State in terms of lowering costs and greater regulation from the centre does not necessarily mean that globalization can be associated with such moves. They argue that there is much room for manoeuvre for national governments in opposing the forces of globalization which shows that although many national governments may have been captured by the globalization thesis governments still have choices to oppose and limit its effects. Thus they point to the considerable differences of approach across different countries to the organization and delivery of social work and social care services which suggest that globalization is not as all-powerful in its effects as some would argue.

Both sets of authors accept that there are profound changes occurring in the world economy which have a significant impact upon the delivery and organization of services. New Labour has largely accepted the globalization thesis and has developed social policy with globalization in mind. As Tony Blair has outlined, for him the globalized world economy is a fact:

> A country has to dismantle barriers to competition and accept the disciplines of the international economy. That has been happening the world over, to varying degrees, in what might be called the first era response to globalisation.
>
> (Blair 1996, p. 118)

New Labour's strategy for welfare is to contain expenditure on social benefits while increasing spending on programmes which directly or indirectly lead to employment. The New Deal is a prime example of this, targeting the young unemployed, single carers and disabled people among others in programmes to place them in the labour market. This approach is underpinned by a strong commitment to use the social security system not as a means to redistribute income from rich to poor, nor as a minimal safety net for the poorest, but as a trampoline to bounce people back into work and, it is argued, inclusion into society. As the Commission on Social Justice (1994, p. 224) which was charged with identifying a radically new approach for the Labour Party in respect of the Welfare State put it: 'The Welfare State must offer a hand-up rather than a handout.'

This approach is meant to carve out a niche for New Labour between what it would argue are the discredited policies of Old Labour, which in its view undermined economic progress through indiscriminate social spending and therefore ignored the realities of globalization, and the Conservative Party, which undermined economic progress with an indiscriminate faith in the market in a headlong rush to embrace globalization.

For those individuals and communities unable to respond to the challenges of globalization who are living in entrenched poverty and experiencing profound social exclusion, a longer-term strategy is more appropriate. The Labour government is attempting to develop a co-ordinated response to poverty and social exclusion through the Social Exclusion Unit within the Cabinet Office (see Chapter 3). However, the Social Exclusion Unit does not have a budget to implement these plans, but will attempt to co-ordinate appropriate government departments to develop policies to tackle social exclusion. Its initial priorities were truancy, street homelessness and neighbourhood renewal. The Unit is taking a long view and suggests that its success should be measured at the end of ten years.

For the users of social work services the commitment to counter social exclusion is welcome but the effects may be less so, particularly as the government is determined to keep tight control over the social security budget. New Labour has become an enthusiastic selectivist targeting help where it believes it to be most deserving and encouraging and requiring work for those whom it considers are able. Peter Mandelson, one of the architects of New Labour's policy, is unwavering in this as he sets out policy for the second term of the Labour government; welfare should be about 'helping people help themselves and widening participation in employment' (Mandelson 2001). An example of this approach relates to disability: the government has introduced tighter controls on eligibility to incapacity benefit (paid to those who were in work and who are now unable to) for disabled people and withdrawing benefit from those who have their own private pension schemes or savings by means testing this benefit. As Lister (1997, p. 7), a critic of New Labour's approach, has argued:

> There has been a subtle shift from arguing that tackling poverty cannot simply be about extra money for those on benefit, a position which can hardly be disputed, to a position that is not about better benefits period.

The primary aim is therefore to create a society which gives primacy to work; those who can must work and if they refuse they will be subject to scrutiny, control and in the final instance a reduction in benefit. This will mean that benefits will become increasingly tied to claimants fulfiling certain conditions set down by government. It may not stop at requiring people to work but can be extended towards any behaviour which the government wishes to shape towards its own vision of propriety. The Crime and Disorder Act 1998 is an example of such an approach; for instance, Anti-Social Behaviour Orders require parents of constantly offending children to attend classes in controlling and parenting their children, while Community Safety Orders can be served on individuals and families requiring them to move from a particular area where they are considered to be involved in violent harassment or antisocial behaviour. Although problems of antisocial behaviour and failure to find or maintain employment are not directly the same, the general policy is to require individuals to meet what New Labour considers to be their duties before the state will respond in recognizing individuals as full citizens.

The difficulties in such an approach can be recognized if the compulsory element of the New Deal is taken into account. This affects the young unemployed 18–24-year-olds and the long-term unemployed (unemployed for two years plus). Thus these groups are required to take up options of employment/education or training in which a refusal may see their benefit payments reduced or stopped in some cases. Although in terms of reducing unemployment the New Deal can be considered a limited success, particularly for those who require little help, this has been achieved at a point of relatively high employment opportunities. However, where the New Deal is less successful is with precisely those groups of people that social workers engage with. Thus those people who experience profound social exclusion and those with 'special needs' do not fare well under the New Deal regime (Millar 2001). Thus to impose a tough policy of benefit reduction on these groups is merely to compound their problems. Although evidence of the consequences of compulsion is limited in the UK there is ample evidence from the USA where similar schemes have operated for a long time and in which the consequences are serious for those affected. Cammisa (1998) suggests a number of problems with compulsion experienced in the USA. These are as follows:

- behaviour of the poorest is subject to regulation, leaving the wealthy to act as they will
- punishment through benefit reduction affects children of those punished, putting them at greater risk
- it reinforces class and race stereotypes as those who are punished come from minorities such as working-class, ethnic minorities, and encourages middle classes to have negative attitudes towards the poor
- can eliminate claimants from their right to welfare; discourages claiming of benefit if subject to punitive treatment
- forces the unemployed into poorly paid and often inappropriate employment
- swaps poverty on benefit for poverty in work.

Single parents or welfare mothers as they are called in the USA are particularly disadvantaged by compelling welfare to work. Research for the American Congress suggests that a quarter maintain their jobs earning as much as they did on welfare, one-half are worse off than being on welfare, and a quarter will be in such severe difficulty that they will have to give up their children or, in trying to keep their families together, they will spend time as homeless people (Katz in Cammisa 1998, p. 121). However, compelling those on welfare benefits into work does not have to be at the forefront of policy as evidence from Scandinavia shows, where similar schemes require the unemployed to engage in work and retraining. The schemes available are underpinned by the unemployed having rights to a wide range of varied and generous schemes which win the consent of the unemployed rather than require their obedience (Etherington 1998). Thus people feel that the available schemes address their needs for retraining rather than the needs of the state for reduced benefit payments.

As New Labour has attempted to respond to the competitive pressures of globalization, it has followed a road which has focused upon investment in welfare for a productivity advantage; this may be a more palatable alternative to one which pursues a low wage, low welfare expenditure route. However, as Deacon *et al.* (1997) argue, the outcome of both strategies is to create a splintered society in which the work rich protected by social insurance benefits, secure working conditions and the income to use private provision where necessary are separated from those who exist on poverty wages or on inadequate means-tested benefits.

New Labour and devolution

Since coming to power, New Labour has followed a policy of regionalization and devolution. Scotland now has its own Parliament as power has transferred to a Scottish Executive, Wales has an assembly coming through the Office of the National Assembly for Wales, and Northern Ireland an assembly through the Northern Ireland Executive. At present it is too early to assess the impact of devolution but as it develops there are likely to be significant variations in the delivery and organization of services to account for the particular needs of the devolved populations (see Drakeford 1998; Kilbane 2000). New Labour would also like to develop regional elected assemblies for England. In terms of independence, Scotland has made greater advances; the Scottish Parliament can raise revenue to fund services it has responsibility for and can legislate on a wide range of non-reserved matters, such as social care and education. However, it has no power over social security, defence, foreign affairs or economic policy which are still controlled by central government. Wales on the other hand has an elected Assembly which has less power than the Scottish Parliament, being unable to raise its own taxation or develop new legislation. The Welsh Assembly can vary and amend central government legislation to respond to local conditions such as the rural nature of Wales and the distinctive requirement to reflect the Welsh language within a bilingual policy towards public life. Devolution is politically a difficult problem for central government and there have been calls for a re-evaluation of the funding of local government services (for example, education and the PSS) through the revenue support grant as it is argued that there are disparities in funding between English authorities and devolved authorities. New Labour has also faced considerable political embarrassment in terms of social policy issues from the Scottish Parliament. For example, the issue of long-term care for older people is being dealt with in a universalist way in Scotland where there is a strong likelihood that the Scottish Labour Party who are in a coalition with the Liberal Democrats will introduce free long-term residential care for those requiring it. The Welsh Assembly has also campaigned for free long-term care for Wales. If the Scottish policy is implemented it will provide a strong impetus for the campaign for free long-term care in England as the current policy reflects a means-tested approach (see Chapter 5).

New Labour's moral agenda

New Labour's approach is to a large extent based upon communitarian approaches to welfare. Although there are many versions of communitarianism, the key concept is the threat to community posed by over-ambitious governments either by the use of the market (by the Right) or the use of the state (by the Left). Both approaches it is argued fragment and break down the social relationships that people develop within local communities (Etzioni 1993). This view harks back to ideas that underpin community care (see Chapter 5), a kind of small town or neighbourhood vision which some would say has been lost but which critics argue has never actually existed. As Bauman (2001, p. 5) suggests, many myths have predominated about the community and reflect an unfulfilled longing: 'In short "community" stands for the kind of world which is not, regrettably, available to us – but which we would dearly wish to inhabit and which we hope to repossess.'

The belief in community and the impact of communitarianism upon New Labour has meant that state action through neighbourhood renewal schemes or the modernizing of local government seeks to chart a precarious course. As noted above, for communitarians too much state involvement in people's lives reduces their own initiative and leads to communities which have weak social attachments; too much state encouragement of the market leads to individuals who remain self-interested, lacking a concern for others, which in turn leads to a breakdown in social bonds and attachments. The purpose of government as New Labour sees it is to rebuild the framework of social relationships in communities, emphasizing the duties and responsibilities which individuals should meet. What New Labour seeks is a society which is cohesive based upon social solidarity in which individual choice is woven into ideas of collective responsibility; thus individuals must be allowed their freedom to act, but not irresponsibly in terms that New Labour defines. Their actions must not ignore majority moral principles which membership of a society requires us to uphold (Jordan 1998).

The communitarian turn by New Labour has been described by Driver and Martell (1997), from which the following model has been extracted. New Labour's social policy moves towards:

- conditionalism
- moralism

- social conservatism
- prescriptivism.

Conditionalism

This places a greater emphasis upon providing rights to welfare in return for a greater exercise of responsibility by members of the community. The New Deal requires young people to take advantage of job offers and retraining while removing their right to benefit if they refuse. This also has implications for organizations; for example, New Labour requires local authorities to act in relation to conditions of service delivery set down by them. If they fail in their duty they are likely to face financial penalties or have their managerial responsibilities removed. Thus a number of local authority children's departments have been subject to special measures where their performance is scrutinized, and some have had their administration of children's services removed, such as Wirral Children's Service.

Moralism

This attempts to develop social cohesion through a return to basic moral values; this can be discerned in the call for maintaining the nuclear family, the importance of work to break the so-called 'dependency culture'. Increasingly the government has also looked towards 'faith communities', involving religious organizations more closely with the Welfare State, particularly in the area of community development and community care through its development of voluntary organizations (Home Office 1998b).

Social conservatism

New Labour has increasingly promoted conservative morality, particularly around parenting and education. The government invocation that poverty is no excuse for failing schools may be welcome as a call for action but not if it forgets the weight of sociological evidence which shows the importance of social background on educational attainment.

Prescriptivism

Contrary to the suggestions of communitarians, New Labour wishes to prescribe the values and morality to which communities should adhere. When the community is invoked it appears that it is the government which seeks to enforce values rather than communities themselves. Thus, rather than values being promoted by the community to meet their concerns, values are prescribed by government. This may be recognized in the enforcement of work upon single parents as a moral good, the admonishment of failing schools or the promotion of 'zero tolerance' within the criminal justice system. Best Value works in similar ways for local authorities where standards of service are prescribed through performance indicators in which local authorities are required to meet these outcomes in particular ways.

New Labour and the PSS

New Labour has attempted to introduce its own version of a 'Third Way' into the PSS. This, following Jordan and Jordan (2000), involves a number of key themes which are necessarily interconnected but for the sake of clarity will be identified separately:

1   breaking down barriers
2   harmonizing policies
3   indicators and targets
4   contracting and quasi-markets
5   public–private partnerships.

Breaking down barriers

New Labour is attempting to open up opportunities for inclusion by reducing the impediments to the participation of the poor in what they consider to be valued means in society, particularly for work. This objective requires local authorities to consult with their communities to consumer research the requirements for services which are valued. This operates at the level of citizens' capacities through policies to reduce social exclusion and at the level of the communities in which the excluded live. Thus money is directed through Single Regeneration Budgets and the New Deal for Communities and is designed to target the most deprived neighbourhoods, bringing together a range of policies and initiatives such as employment, health and education action zones. For example, health action zones bring together all those government agencies concerned with health development, requiring them to work towards health improvement and target particular groups at risk of health exclusion such as young people leaving care, or teenage mothers. This policy however echoes the New Deal for the unemployed in that it is not designed for physical renewal as such but for developing better opportunities for local people and forms of attitude change and behaviour modification. For example, the Sure Start Programme which is designed to support young families in poverty with advice, guidance and training around parenting.

Harmonizing policies

This refers to New Labour's attempt to bring together different government and local government agencies around particular problems to ensure consistency and co-ordination of response. The setting up of Health Care Trusts is one such initiative which seeks to bring health and personal social services together to plan and deliver social care for those people leaving hospital. Likewise the Social Exclusion Unit is one such co-ordinating body which seeks to harmonize the approaches of different governmental and non-governmental bodies to deliver co-ordinated policies for a specifically identified group such as care leavers or rough sleepers.

Indicators and targets

We have identified this approach in relation to children's services around the National Assessment Framework and Quality Protects (Chapter 6). This creates a powerful tool for central government and its appointees within regional bodies to monitor failing performance and praise success. It thus gives power to the centre to name and shame local authorities which are failing to meet the agreed standards and criteria and hold staff to account for their own work through regulation and control of professional work. The Social Care Council, when it finally comes on stream, will act to regulate the behaviour of social work and social care professionals. As Jordan and Jordan (2000, p. 28) bleakly comment, this will further limit the professional discretion and creativity of workers: 'Social work is not an art or even a science, but an instrument of ministerial will.'

Contracting and quasi-markets

The retention of quasi-markets in community care and their further development within children's services requires local authorities and the independent sector to be continually trimming operations to meet the requirements of economy, efficiency and effectiveness. The use of Best Value is instructive here as the PSS are brought under a regime which covers the whole of local government, something they were immune from although not from the quasi-market process under the NHSCCA 1990.

Public–private partnerships

The PSS will increasingly be drawn towards developing investment in new buildings and services through public–private partnerships. We have already highlighted some of these problems in relation to the NHS and the principles will remain in relation to the PSS. Under Best Value, local authorities are being encouraged to enter into long-term relationships with private providers where they can prove that gains in terms of efficiency and effectiveness can be achieved. Likewise asylum seekers are now also part of this process with private providers supplying accommodation and support services to such service users. Consequently private providers may well be brought in to manage so-called failing authorities within the PSS.

Conclusion

This chapter has shown the way in which the PSS has responded to the important changes which have occurred over the past twenty years. It has highlighted the differences in approach between the immediate post-Seebohm organization of social services and its change following the NHSCCA 1990. It has recognized that New Labour has attempted to forge a different path from that of previous Labour administrations and has done this to differentiate itself from what it considers to be the outdated policies of Old Labour. In achieving success within the party this policy has challenged many of the values of the post-war generation of Labour activists and politicians who saw in the development of a Welfare State a path to socialism. Finally, current policy towards the PSS has been outlined with a discussion of some alternative strategies.

New Labour is actively reconstructing the Welfare State and promises as radical a shake up as the previous Conservative administration attempted. The implications of New Labour's Third Way for those whom the PSS work with may be bleak in a world where the rights to services become increasingly tied in with responsibilities to the state. These responsibilities increase in scope and reach, affecting not only service users but also service providers as well. Organizations such as social services departments which are unable to deliver the New Labour vision are likely to be subject to greater regulation or be replaced by outside bodies both public and private. In redrawing the landscape of the PSS we have seen a further encouragement to be innovative and entrepreneurial so that local government resembles more the operations of a medium-scale corporation. In addition, PSS functions previously held by local authorities are hived off to outside agencies such as inspection to regional care commissions and much of social care to Care Trusts, further reducing the influence of local authorities in the delivery and monitoring of services.

The current government clearly believes that the PSS has failed in many respects to provide adequate community and childcare services. Not surprisingly the current minister responsible for PSS, John Hutton, has no sentimental attachment to the previous structures that have delivered community care and children's services: 'We can't lock into a particular way of delivering service just because that's the historic way that service has been delivered' (Neate 2000).

Thus just as social care merges with the health service so Hutton sees a future where children's services may well merge with the education service, as indeed some already have. As important as organizational change is in meeting new challenges to social work and social care, the distinctive contribution of the PSS may well be lost. One of the reasons for reorganizing the PSS departments in the first place was to provide a co-ordinated social work and social care service which would have the political and organizational power to create universal welfare services with local authorities (see Chapter 2). Organizational change may also mask the sustained underfunding of the PSS which, even with modest increases, has resulted in significant overspending by local authorities to meet government requirements.

Social work and social care is likely to experience further change over the term of the Labour government in which local authorities' responsibility for delivering PSS may all but disappear. The strong working practices and service delivery which has been a constant feature of PSS departments and which is consistently made apparent by the reports of the Audit Commission and the SSI do not grab the headlines in the same way as the admitted mistakes of a minority of local authorities and social workers in failing to care adequately for children or adults in the community. It remains to be seen whether modernization of the PSS will be able to deal with the complex task of delivering PSS any more effectively than the previous organizational regime.

Key points

- The Welfare State has been restructured due to changes in the social, political and economic environment.
- The PSS is in turn being restructured which may lead to its disappearance in organizational terms.
- New Labour's policy agenda targets work to combat social exclusion.
- New Labour has a strong moral agenda which may lead to the further marginalizing of service users of the PSS.

Guide to further reading

Powell, M. (ed.) (1999) *New Labour, New Welfare State? The 'Third Way' in British Social Policy*, Bristol: Policy Press, is an excellent summary of New Labour's approach to social policy. To understand New Labour's position prior to becoming a government the Borrie Commission (1994) *Social Justice: Strategies for National Renewal – The Report on the Commission for Social Justice*, London: Vintage, is essential. Toynbee, P. and Walker, D. (2001) *Did Things Get Better? An Audit of Labour's Successes and Failures*, London: Penguin, provides a useful if sometimes uncritical account of New Labour's first administration.

Glossary

Anti-discriminatory practice: An approach to social work practice which seeks to understand the basis of oppression and discrimination in society through social divisions of age, race, sexuality, class and disability, and works to eradicate their discriminatory consequences in society. This requires social workers to work to eliminate such discrimination and oppression in their own practice, social work organizations and the institutions of the Welfare State.

Anti-racism: An analysis which explains racism as deep-seated within the institutions of society. Applied to social policy, it seeks to explain the oppression experienced by black people as a result of the way racism, as a dominant aspect of British culture, has permeated all the institutions of the Welfare State.

Best Value: Refers to the process by which government will require continuing and improved performance of local authorities in the management and delivery of local authority services. This will be measured through Best Value performance indicators, the main focus being upon maintaining competition within the mixed economy of locally based services.

Care Trust: Organization set up within the NHS to integrate the work of health and the PSS in the delivery of social care through, for example, pooling of budgets and integrated working.

Citizens' Charter: Introduced by the previous Conservative government in an attempt to introduce elements of consumer choice to users of the Welfare State. Thus it has required a range of welfare services to publish statistics on their performance against set criteria, such as league tables in education which are supposed to allow parents to judge one school's performance against another's to decide to which school they should send their children.

Citizenship: Most famously used by T.H. Marshall when he outlined the three aspects of citizenship as civil rights (freedom of the individual, equality before the law), political rights (freedom of association, right to vote) and social rights (e.g. rights to a minimum income, basic health care). As Chapter 7 points out, this is a contested subject in which different political ideologies influence different definitions as either maximalist (to include social rights) or minimalist (to limit the range of rights provided by the state to the civil and political sphere).

Communitarianism: A political philosophy which criticizes individualistic approaches to society. Suggests that societies shape and mould individuals' approach to such issues as morality, rights and responsibilities rather than the actions of individuals. Popularized by Etzioni (1993) but has also been developed more systematically by a range of political philosophers, e.g. Taylor, Walzer and Sandel (Mulhall and Swift 1994).

Dependency: Describes the over-reliance on state welfare, which is said to prevent people from making an effort to support themselves. Originally used by those on the political Right, it has now been increasingly adopted by New Labour in its reform of the social security system, particularly in relation to single parents and the long-term unemployed.

Equality of opportunity: Used either to emphasize giving everyone an equal opportunity to compete in an unequal society, or to emphasize equality of outcome, equality of opportunity attempts to promote an equal society by equalizing the outcomes achieved by individuals so that they are valued equally.

Eugenics: Developed in the late nineteenth century, eugenics heavily influenced many welfare reformers both within the COS and the Fabian Society. Based upon a 'science' of heredity, eugenics asserts that human beings inherit characteristics which determine their subsequent life history. Thus social problems such as crime, for example, are caused by those who are biologically disposed towards them. Recent examples can be found in the work of Charles Murray (see Chapter 3) who asserts that the poor educational achievement and high dependence on welfare by black Americans can be explained by their inadequate stock of intelligence genes.

Exit and voice: Used to denote respectively the power consumers have to exit from one service to the next if they are dissatisfied with the service they receive or the power citizens have in voicing their preferences for particular services within a participatory framework.

Institutionalization: The process by which large numbers of people (e.g. those with mental health problems or learning disabilities) were placed in large hospitals/asylums. It can also refer to the damaging experience of living in such places characterized by isolation, dull routine and lack of personal freedom.

Means test: A procedure mostly used within the social security system to limit the distribution of benefits and services to an identified group of individuals whose income and/or assets fall below a specified level. This is increasingly being used in community care services to limit the levels of domiciliary and social care available.

National Assessment Frameworks: Sets out guidance for the assessment of needs across a variety of service user groups (e.g. in relation to children and older people).

New Deal: One of the key policy initiatives of the current Labour government. It uses a 'windfall tax' taken from excess profits of the privatized utilities to create training and work opportunities for identified groups excluded from the labour market.

New Labour: Label used by the ruling group within the Labour Party to distance itself from the values and policies of 'Old Labour', seen as out of date and unelectable. One of the key issues here was the changing of Labour's constitution to remove nationalization as one of the main aims of the party.

New Right: Powerful ideology of the 1980s, heavily influenced by ideas of nineteenth-century free market economics and traditional notions of morality. It represents a belief in the unfettered use of markets and a minimum of state involvement in the economy, coupled with a powerful state which maintains law and order and so-called traditional values of family, church and nation.

Normalization: Describes the process by which people, who are usually denied opportunities for full participation in society, such as people with learning disabilities, can be enabled to maximize their participation and acquire valued roles in society.

Performance indicators: Attempts to create 'objective' measures of service performance which can be assessed to monitor outcomes of service delivery.

Privatization: The process by which state-controlled utilities and services are sold off to the private sector. In the PSS this has meant, among other things, local authority residential homes for older people being sold to the private sector.

Public–private partnerships: Mostly financial partnerships between the state and the private sector used to fund investment in the Welfare State, these have been used falteringly within the NHS to build new hospitals, and are likely to expand into other areas of welfare.

Selectivism: The process of allocating welfare service or benefits by selecting the most 'needy' through an income or means test, closely aligned with, but not the same as, targeting.

Social division: Used in this book to identify the way in which the Welfare State divides different social groups, for example, women or black people, into positions of inferiority through a discriminatory process of access and allocation of welfare.

Social exclusion: The process by which people are prevented from participation in society which takes into account the range of opportunities, access to services and social networks which people rely upon to make a valued life for themselves.

Social work values: The principles that should guide social workers in their practice.

Standard Spending Assessment (SSA): The method used by central government to determine the level of grant to be given to local authorities from the Revenue Support Grant. The assessment is a complex weighting of social and geographical factors said to reflect the needs of local areas, and is used to determine the amounts of money going to individual services controlled by local authorities such as the PSS.

State, the: At its basic level, refers to the institutions in society through which governments rule and influence the behaviour of populations (e.g. those institutions involved in welfare such as social security, education and the family).

Targeting: The concentration of welfare benefits and services upon particular groups identified as being in greatest need. For example, the New Deal targets its service towards the long-term unemployed, single parents and people with disabilities.

Third Way: An ideology which is committed to repudiate both individualistic approaches to politics and the Welfare State such as the New Right and traditional collectivist approaches based upon Fabianism and Social Democracy. In respect to welfare it seeks to use the Welfare State to create opportunities for individual advancement and social cohesion.

Universalism: The principle of providing welfare benefits and services to the whole population based on their equal rights as citizens.

Welfare pluralism: The way in which welfare can be produced and consumed through statutory and non-statutory ways; current community care arrangements favour a welfare pluralist approach.

Some useful websites and journals

These websites were operational at the time of going to press, but because of the nature of the Internet, they may move to new addresses or no longer be in operation. For those new to the web a useful guide has been published by Stuart Stein (1999) *Learning, Teaching and Researching on the Internet: A Practical Guide for Social Scientists*, London: Longman.

Websites

http://www.sosig.ac.uk/
This is the Social Science Information Gateway; this facility provides links to over 1,000 UK and worldwide social science resources. You can search for topics by entering keywords into its search facility. Also provides a useful introduction for social workers in using the site.

http://www.nisw.org.uk/
Website address for the National Institute for Social Work in the UK; along with its own published reports (some of which you can find in shortened versions called Findings) they also host the worldwide web resources for social work, which provide an enormous range of information on national and international organizations, services and research across the range of social work.

http://www.open.gov.uk/
This provides access to all government departments, local authorities and many other official agencies. It also provides a search index of other central and local government sites.

http://www.cre.gov.uk
Excellent website for Commission for Racial Equality provides a wealth of information on the law and useful case examples of successful actions in the courts by the CRE.

http://www.eoc.gov.ukl
Another excellent site for Equal Opportunities Commission provides detailed and comprehensive information in relation to research on women's pay, successful court actions and the law.

http://www.jrf.org.uk
This is the site for the Joseph Rowntree Trust which funds research into social policy. It is particularly strong on social work and is an excellent source of information on research. Click into their Findings section.

http://www.community-care.co.uk
This is the website for the magazine *Community Care*, a journal written for the social work profession. It provides up-to-date news, comment, short articles and debate on an extensive range of social work issues.

http://www.workhouses.co.uk
Take a virtual tour of a workhouse, access contemporary accounts from inmates, journalists and novelists. Add your own comments to the site upon the impact of the workhouse within British social history. Songs, poems and other documents are all included. A favourite site for students.

http://www.audit-commission.gov.uk
The Audit Commission provides part of the government's inspection service and is worth accessing for the many reports on the operation of the personal social services within local authorities. Provides much basic information on the performance of local authority social service departments.

http://www.disabilityalliance.org
Provides a wealth of information on all aspects of disability particularly in relation to social security and the personal social services.

http://www.dss.gov.uk/
The Department of Social Security has provided an excellent website from which you can access a range of information on the social security system. Of particular interest is a history of the social security system, with archive material on the Beveridge Report and contemporary views of the social security system at different historical periods.

Journals

Many students seem put off using academic journals and only discover their usefulness when they are near completion of their studies. Journals can provide useful summaries of often complex arguments but also provide up-to-date research material. Remember: most books, even with the speed of publishing now made possible by new technology, can still be up to eighteen months old. All journals are now made available via the internet and examples of full text material can usually be downloaded. Here is a brief list:

Ageing and Society
Benefits
British Journal of Social Work
Child and Family Social Work
Critical Social Policy
Disability and Society
Economy and Society
Journal of Social Policy
Journal of European Social Policy
Journal of European Social Work
Policy and Politics
Practice
Social Policy and Administration

There are many more. Browse around your journals library and you will always find something of relevance for your studies.

References

Acheson, D. (1998) *Independent Enquiry into Inequalities in Health*, London: HMSO.

Adams, R. (1996) *The Personal Social Services*, London: Longman.

Adams, R. (1998*)* *Quality Social Work*, London: Macmillan.

Adelman, I. and Bradshaw, J. (1999) *Children in Poverty: An Analysis of the Family Resources Survey 1994/95*, York: York University and Social Policy Research Unit.

Alcock, P. (1996) *Social Policy in Britain*, London: Macmillan.

Alcock, P. and Pearson, S. (1999) Raising the poverty plateau: the impact of means tested rebates from local authority charges on low income households', *Journal of Social Policy*, 28(3), pp. 497–516.

Alibhai-Brown,Y. (1993) 'Social workers need race training, not hysteria', *Independent*, 11 August.

Andrews, G. and Phillips, D. (2000) 'Private residential care for older persons: local impacts of care in the community reforms in England and Wales', *Social Policy and Administration*, 34(2), pp. 206–222.

Annual Abstract of Statistics (1997) London: HMSO.

Association of Directors of Social Services and Commission for Racial Equality (1978) *Multi-Racial Britain: The Social Services Response*, London: ADSS/CRE.

Audit Commission (1986) *Making a Reality of Community Care*, London: HMSO.

Audit Commission (1994a) *Taking Stock; Progress with Care in the Community*, London: HMSO.

Audit Commission (1994b) *Seen But Not Heard: Coordinating Community Child Health and Social Services for Children in Need*, London: HMSO.

Audit Commission (2000) *Charging with Care: How Councils Charge for Home Care*, London: HMSO.

Baistow, K. (1995) 'Some paradoxes of empowerment', *Critical Social Policy*, Winter (2), pp. 32–46.

Baistow, K., Hetherington, R., Spriggs, A. and Yelloly, M. (1996) *Parents Speaking: Anglo-French Perceptions of Child Welfare Interventions?*, London: Brunel University College.

Baldock, J. (1997) 'The personal social services and community care', in Alcock, P. *et al.* (1997) *The Students' Companion to Social Policy*, Oxford: Blackwell.

Baldwin, S. and Lunt, N. (1996) *Local Authority Charging Policies for Community Care*,York: Joseph Rowntree Foundation.

Ball, R., Heafey, M. and King, D. (2001) 'Private finance initiative – a good deal for the public purse or a drain on future generations?', *Policy and Politics*, 29(1), pp. 95–108.

Barclay, P. (1982) *Social Workers: Their Role and Tasks*, London: Bedford Press.

Barnes, C., Mercer, G. and Shakespeare, T. (1999) *Exploring Disability: A Sociological Introduction*, Cambridge: Polity Press.

Barnes, M. (1997) *Care, Communities and Citizens*, London: Longman.

Barnes, M. (1999) 'Users as citizens: collective action and the local governance of welfare', *Social Policy and Administration*, March(1), pp. 73–90.

Barry, M. and Hallett, C. (1998) *Social Exclusion and Social Work*, Lyme Regis, Dorset: Russell House.

Bates, J., Pugh, R. and Thompson, N. (1997) *Protecting Children: Challenges and Change*, Aldershot: Arena.

Batsleer, J. and Humphries, B. (2000) 'Welfare, exclusion and political agency', in Batsleer, J. and Humphries, B. *Welfare, Exclusion and Political Agency*, London: Routledge.

Bauman, Z. (2001) *Community: Seeking Safety in an Insecure World*, Cambridge: Polity Press.

Bebbington, A. and Kelly, A. (1995) 'Expenditure planning in the personal social services', *Journal of Social Policy*, 24(3).

Bebbington, A. and Miles, J. (1989) 'The background of children who enter local authority care', *British Journal of Social Work*, 19(5), pp. 349–368.

Beishon, S., Modood, T. and Virdee, S. (1998) *Ethnic Minority Families*, London: Policy Studies Institute.

Bell, D. (1993) *Communitarianism and its Critics*, Oxford: Clarendon Press.

Beresford, P. and Turner, M. (1997) *Its Our Welfare: Report of the Citizens' Commission on the Future of the Welfare State*, London: National Institute of Social Work.

Berridge, D. (1997) *Foster Care: A Research Review*, London: HMSO.

Berridge, D. and Brodie, I. (1998) *Children's Homes Revisited*, London: Jessica Kingsley.

Bilson, A. and Barker, R. (1995) 'Parental contact with children fostered and in residential care after the Children Act 1989', *British Journal of Social Work*, 25, pp. 367–381.

Blair, T. (1996) *New Britain: My Vision of a Young Country*, London: Fourth Estate.

Blair, T. (1997) 'Why we must help those excluded from society', *Independent*, 8 December.

Blakemore, K. and Drake, R. (1996) *Understanding Equal Opportunity Policies*, Hemel Hempstead: Prentice Hall/Harvester Wheatsheaf.

Booth, T. and Booth, W. (1994) *Parenting under Pressure*, Buckingham: Open University Press.

Boyne, G.A., (1999) *Managing Local Services: From CCT to Best Value*, London: Frank Cass.

Boyson, R. (ed.) (1971) *Down with the Poor*, London: Churchill Press.

Brandon, M., Thoburn, J., Lewis, A. and Way, A. (1999) 'Safeguarding children with the Children Act', in D. Platt (2000) 'Refocusing children's services: evaluation of an initial assessment process', *Child and Family Social Work*, 6, pp. 139–148.

Brown, C. (1984) *Black and White Britain*, London: Heinemann.

Brown, J. (1990) 'The focus on single mothers', in Murray, C. *The Emerging British Underclass*, London: IEA.

Brown, J. (1995) 'Can social work empower?', in Hugman, R. and Smith, D. *Ethical Issues in Social Work*, London: Routledge.

Butt, J. (1994) *Same Service or Equal Service?*, London: HMSO.

Byrne, D. (1999) *Social Exclusion,* Buckingham: Open University Press.

Cammisa, A. (1998) *From Rhetoric to Reform? Welfare Policy in American Politics*, Oxford: Westview Press.

CCETSW (1995) *Requirements and Regulations for the Diploma in Social Work* (Paper 30 revised), London: CCETSW.

Central Statistical Office (1994) *General Household Survey*, London: HMSO.

Central Statistical Office (1996) *Social Trends*, London: HMSO.

Central Statistical Office (2000) *Social Trends*, London: HMSO.

Chand, A. (2000) 'The over-representation of Black children in the child protection system: possible causes, consequences and solutions', *Child and Family Social Work*, 5, pp. 67–77.

Charles, N. (2000) *Feminism, The State and Social Policy*, London: Macmillan.

Chetwynd, M., Ritchie, J., Reith, L. and Howard, M. (1996) *The Cost of Care: The Impact of Charging Policy on the Lives of Disabled People*, York: Joseph Rowntree Trust.

Clark, C. (1998) 'Self-determination and paternalism in community care', *British Journal of Social Work*, 28, pp. 387–402.

Clarke, J. (1980) 'Social Democratic delinquents and Fabian families', in National Deviancy Conference (ed.) *Permissiveness and Control*, London: Macmillan.

Clarke, J. (1993) *A Crisis in Care? Challenges to Social Work*, London: Sage.

Clarke, J., Cochrane, A. and Smart, C. (1987) *Ideologies of Welfare: From Dreams to Disillusion*, London: Hutchinson.

Coard, B. (1971) *How West Indian Children are Made Educationally Subnormal*, London: New Beacon.

Commission on Social Justice (1994) *Social Justice*, London: Vintage.

Community Care (2001) 'Councils seek meeting with ministers over budget crisis', *Community Care Journal*, 1 February.

Corby, B. (2000) The impact of public enquiries', in Crimmens, D. and Pitts, J. *Positive Residential Practice: Learning the Lessons of the 1990s*, Lyme Regis: Russell House.

Corby, B. and Millar, M. (1997) 'A parents' view of partnership', in Bates, J. *et al. Protecting Children: Challenges and Change*, op. cit., pp. 75–88.

Cosis-Brown, H. (1998) *Social Work and Sexuality*, London: Macmillan.

Creighton, S. J. (1995) 'Fatal child abuse – how preventable is it?', *Child Abuse Review*, 4, pp. 318–328.

Crimmens, D. and Pitts, J. (2000) *Positive Residential Practice: Learning the Lessons of the 1990s*, Lyme Regis, Dorset: Russell House.

Croft, S. and Beresford, P. (1997) 'Service users' perspectives', in Davies, M. (ed.) *The Blackwell Companion to Social Work*, Oxford: Blackwell, pp. 272–279.

Crompton, R. (1993) *Class and Stratification*, Cambridge: Polity Press.

Dalley, G. (1997) *Ideologies of Caring – Rethinking Community and Collectivism*, London: Macmillan (2nd edn).

Dartington Social Research Unit (1995) *Child Protection: Messages from Research*, London: HMSO.

Davies, C. (2000) 'The demise of professional self-regulation: a moment to mourn?, in Lewis, G., Gewirtz, S. and Clarke, J. *Rethinking Social Policy*, London: Sage.

Davis, A. (1996) 'Women and the personal social services' in Hallett, C. (ed.) *Women and Social Policy*, London: Prentice Hall/Harvester Wheatsheaf.

Deacon, B., Hulse, M. and Stubbs, P. (1997) *Global Social Policy: International Organizations and the Future of Welfare*, London: Sage.

Dean, H. and Taylor-Gooby, P. (1992) *Dependency Culture: The Explosion of a Myth*, Hemel Hempstead: Harvester Wheatsheaf.

Dearden, C. and Becker, S. (2000) 'Young carers: needs, rights and assessments', in Department of Health *The Child's World: Assessing Children in Need*, London: Department of Health.

Dennis, N. (1993) *Rising Crime and the Dismembered Family: How Conformist Intellectuals have Campaigned Against Common Sense*, London: IEA.

Dennis, N. and Erdos, G. (1992) *Families Without Fatherhood*, London: IEA.

Department of the Environment, Transport and the Regions (1998) *Improving Local Services Through Best Value*, London: HMSO.

Department of Health and Social Security (1975a) *Better Services for the Mentally Handicapped*, Cmnd 4683, London: HMSO.

Department of Health and Social Security (1975b) *Better Services for the Mentally Ill*, Cmnd 6233, London: HMSO.

Department of Health and Social Security (1981) *Growing Older*, Cmnd 8173, London: HMSO.

Department of Health and Social Security (1987) *The Law on Child Care and Family Services*, London: HMSO.

Department of Health and Social Security (1988) *Working Together. A Guide to Arrangements for Inter Agency Co-operation for the Protection of Children from Abuse*, London: HMSO.

Department of Health (1989) *Caring for People: Community Care in the Next Decade and Beyond*, Cm 849, London: HMSO.

Department of Health (1991) *Patterns and Outcomes in Child Placement*, London: HMSO.

Department of Health (1998) *Quality Protects; A Framework for Action and Objectives for Social Services for Children*, London: Department of Health.

Department of Health (1999a) *Modernising Social Services, Promoting Independence, Improving Protection, Raising Standards*, London: Department of Health.

Department of Health (1999b) *The Personal Social Services Performance Assessment Framework*, Local Authority Circular, London.

Department of Health (1999c) *Me, Survive out There?*, London: Department of Health.

Dowling, M. (1998) *Poverty*, Birmingham: Venture Press.

Drakeford, M. (1998) 'Health and social care services and the National Assembly for Wales', *Research Policy and Planning*, 17(2), pp. 1–8.

Driver, S. and Martell, L. (1997) 'New Labour's communitarians', *Critical Social Policy*, August, 17(3).

Edwards, R. and Duncan, S. (1997) 'Supporting the family: lone mothers, paid work and the underclass debate', *Critical Social Policy*, 17(4), pp. 29–49.

Ellis, K. (1993) *Squaring the Circle: User and Carer Participation in Needs Assessment*, York: Joseph Rowntree Foundation.

Ellis, K., Davis, A. and Rummery, K. (1999) 'Needs assessment, street-level bureaucracy and the new community care', *Social Policy and Administration*, 33(3), pp. 262–280.

English, D., Wingard, T., Marshall, D., Orme, M. and Orme, A. (2000) 'Alternative responses to child protective services: emerging issues and concerns', *Child Abuse and Neglect*, 24, pp. 375–388.

Erskine, A. (1997) 'The approaches and methods of social policy', in Alcock, P. *et al. The Students' Companion to Social Policy*, Oxford: Blackwell.

Etherington, D. (1998) 'From welfare to work in Denmark: an alternative to free market policies', *Policy and Politics*, 26(2), pp. 145–163.

Etzioni, A. (1993) *The Spirit of Community*, New York: Basic Books.

Fairclough, N. (2000) *New Labour New Language*, London: Routledge.

Farmer, E. and Owen, M. (eds) (1995) *Child Protection Practice: Private Risks and Public Remedies*, London: HMSO.

Fawcett, B. (2000) *Feminist Perspectives on Disability*, Harlow: Prentice Hall.

Field, F. (1989) *Losing Out: The Emergence of Britain's 'Underclass'*, Oxford: Blackwell.

Field, F. (1997) *Stakeholder Welfare*, London: IEA.

Foucault, M. (1977) *Discipline and Punish*, London: Allen Lane.

Fox-Harding, L. (1996) *Family, State and Social Policy*, London: Macmillan.

Fox-Harding, L. (1997) *Perspectives in Child Care Policy*, London: Longman (2nd edn).

Frost, N. and Stein, M. (1989) *The Politics of Child Welfare*, London: Harvester Wheatsheaf.

George, M. (1996) 'Figure it out', *Community Care*, 1–7 August, Special feature, From Cradle to Grave, pp. i–viii.

George, V. and Wilding, P. (1994) *Welfare and Ideology*, Hemel Hempstead: Harvester Wheatsheaf.

Giarchi, G. and Abbott, P. (1997) 'Old age in Europe', in Spybey, T. (ed.) *Britain in Europe: An Introduction to Sociology*, London: Routledge.

Gibbons, J. S. (1997) 'Relating outcomes to objectives in child protection policy', in Parton, N. (ed.) *Child Protection and Family Support: Tensions, Contradictions and Possibilities*, London: Routledge. pp. 78–91.

Gibbons, J. S., Gallagher, B. and Bell, C. (1995) *Operating the Child Protection System*, London: HMSO.

Giddens, A. (1998) *The Third Way: The Renewal of Social Democracy*, Cambridge: Polity.

Giddens, A. (2001) *Sociology*, Cambridge: Polity (4th edn).

Glyn, S. and Oxborrow, J. (1976) *Inter War Britain: An Economic and Social History*, London: Allen and Unwin.

Gordon, D., Adelman, L., Ashworth, K., Bradshaw, J., Levitas, R., Middleton, S., Pantazis, C., Patzios, D., Payne, S., Townsend, P. and Williams, J. (2000) *Poverty and Social Exclusion in Britain*, York: Joseph Rowntree Foundation.

Griffiths Report (1988) *Community Care; An Agenda for Action*, London: HMSO.

Guardian, (2001) 'Happily ever after', Jobs and Money, 17 March.

Harris, J. (1993) *Private Lives and Public Spirit: Britain 1870–1914*, London: Penguin.

Harris, J. (1999) 'State social work and citizenship in Britain: from clientelism to consumerism', *British Journal Of Social Work*, 29, pp. 915–937.

Henwood, M., Wistow, G. and Robinson, J. (1996) 'Halfway there? Policy, politics and outcomes', *Community Care, Social Policy and Administration*, 30(1), pp. 39–53.

Hetherington, R., Cooper, A., Smith, P. and Wilford, G. (1997) *Protecting Children: Messages from Europe*, Lyme Regis, Dorset: Russell House.

Hill, M. (2000a) 'Conclusions; the future of local authority social services', in Hill, M. (ed.) *Local Authority Social Services: An Introduction*, Oxford: Blackwell.

Hill, M. (ed.) (2000b) *Local Authority Social Services: An Introduction*, Oxford: Blackwell.

Hirst, J. (1997a) 'Taking a long-term view', *Community Care*, 27 March–2 April.

Hirst, J. (1997b) 'Pay for today', *Community Care*, 5–11 June, p. 14.

HMSO (1991) *The Citizen's Charter*, Cmnd 1599, London: HMSO.

HMSO (1985) *House of Commons' Select Committee on the Social Services*, London: HMSO.

HMSO (1996) *House of Commons' Select Committee on Health, Long Term Care: Future Provision and Funding*, London: HMSO.

Holman, R. (1993) *New Deal for Social Welfare*, Oxford: Lion.

Home Office (1998a) *Supporting Families*, London, Home Office.

Home Office (1998b) *Compact: Getting it Right Together*, London, Home Office.

Howarth, C., Kenway, P., Palmer, G. and Miorelli, R. (1999) *Monitoring Poverty and Social Exclusion*, York: Joseph Rowntree/New Policy Institute.

Hughes, B. and Mtezuka, M. (1992) 'Social work and older women: where have all the older women gone?', in Langan, M. and Day, L. *Women, Oppression and Social Work: Issues in Anti-discriminatory Practice*, London: Routledge.

Hughes, G. and Mooney, G. (1998) 'Community', in Hughes, G. (ed.) *Imagining Welfare Futures*, London: Routledge.

Jack, R. (ed.) (1998) *Residential versus Community Care*, London: Macmillan.

Jeffries, A. and Muller, W. (1997) 'Implementing social welfare policy in Europe', in Spybey, T. *Britain in Europe*, London: Routledge.

Jenkins, S. (1995) *Accountable to None*, London: Penguin.

Johnson, N. (1999) 'The personal social services and community care', in Powell, M. (ed.) *New Labour New Welfare State*, Bristol: Policy Press.

Joint Reviews of Local Authorities' Social Services (1997) *Reviewing Social Services*, London: Department of Health/Audit Commission.

Joint Reviews of Local Authorities' Social Services (2000) *Promising Prospects*, London: Department of Health/Audit Commission.

Jones, C. (1996) 'Anti-intellectualism and the peculiarities of British social work education', in Parton, N. (ed.) *Social Theory, Social Change and Social Work*, London: Routledge.

Jordan, B. (1984) *Invitation to Social Work*, Oxford: Martin Robertson.

Jordan, B. (1997) 'Partnership, child protection and family support: trying to square the circle', in Parton, N. (ed.) *Child Protection and Family Support*, London: Routledge.

Jordan, B. (1998) *The New Politics of Welfare: Social Justice in a Global Context*, London: Sage.

Jordan, B. and Jordan, C. (2000) *Social Work and the Third Way: Tough Loves as Social Policy*, London: Sage.

Jordan, M. (1997) 'Risk assessment in residential child care', in Bates, J., Pugh, R. and Thompson, N. *Protecting Children: Challenges and Change*, Aldershot: Arena, pp. 229–236.

Kahan, B. (1994) *Growing up in Groups*, London: NISW.

Kempson, E. (1996) *Life on a Low Income*, York: Joseph Rowntree Foundation.

Khan, P. and Dominelli, L. (2000) 'The impact of globalization on social work in the UK', *European Journal of Social Work*, 3(2). pp. 95–108.

Kilbane, M. (2000) 'Issues and debates: devolution in Northern Ireland', *Research Policy and Planning*, 18(1), pp. 1–3.

Knapp, M., Hardy, B. and Forder, J. (2001) 'Commissioning for quality: ten years of social care markets in England', *Journal of Social Policy*, 30, Part 2, pp. 283–307.

Labour Party (2001) *Ambitions for Britain*, London: Labour Party.

Lamb, B. and Layzell, S. (1995) *Disabled in Britain: Counting on Community Care*, London: Scope.

Lane, D. (2000) 'Often ignored: obvious messages for a safe workforce', in Crimmens, D. and Pitts, J. *Positive Residential Practice: Learning the Lessons of the 1990s*, Lyme Regis, Dorset: Russell House.

Langan, M. (2000) 'Social services: managing the third way', in Clarke, J., Gewitz, S. and Mclaughlin, E. *New Managerialism New Welfare?*, London: Sage.

Langan, M. and Day, L. (1993) *Women, Oppression and Social Work*, London: Routledge.

Langan, M. and Ostner, I. (1991) 'Gender and welfare: towards a comparative framework', in Room, G. (ed.) *Towards a European Welfare State?*, Bristol: SAUS.

Lavalette, M. and Mooney, G. (2000) *Class Struggle and Social Welfare*, London: Routledge.

Law, I. (1996) *Racism, Ethnicity and Social Policy*, Hemel Hempstead: Prentice Hall/Harvester Wheatsheaf.

Levitas, R. (1998) *The Inclusive Society? Social Exclusion and New Labour*, Basingstoke: Macmillan.

Levy, A. and Kahan, B. (1991) *The Pindown Experience and the Protection of Children: The Report of the Staffordshire Child Care Inquiry 1990*, Stafford: Staffordshire County Council.

Lewis, J. (2001) 'Family change and lone parents as a social problem', in May, M., Page, R. and Brundson, E. *Understanding Social Problems; Issues in Social Policy*, Oxford: Blackwell.

Lewis, J., Beenstock, P. and Bovell, V. (1995) 'The community care changes: unresolved tensions in policy and issues in implementation', *Journal of Social Policy*, 24(1), pp. 73–94.

Lister, R. (1997) 'From fractured Britain to One Nation?: The policy options for welfare reform', paper delivered to the Annual Conference of the Social Policy Association, University of Lincolnshire and Humberside, July 1997, pp. 1–15.

Lister, R. (1998) 'In from the margins: citizenship, inclusion and exclusion', in Barry, M. and Hallett, C. *Social Exclusion and Social Work: Issues in Theory and Practice*, Lyme Regis, Dorset: Russell House.

Little, M. (1997) 'The re-focusing of children's services: the contribution of research', in Parton, N. (ed.) *Child Protection and Family Support*, London: Routledge.

Luthra, M. (1997) *Britain's Black Population*, Aldershot: Arena.

Lymberry, M. (1998) 'Care management and professional autonomy: the impact of community care legislation on social work with older people', *British Journal of Social Work*, 28, pp. 863–878.

Lymberry, M. (2000) 'Evaluation: the lost dimension of community care', *Research Policy and Planning*, 18(3), pp. 1–11.

Mandelson, P. (2001) 'Ambition and New Labour', *Observer* 6 May.

Marchant, C. (1995) 'Home of our own', *Community Care*, 6–11 January, pp. 14–15.

Meacher, M. (1972) *Taken for a Ride*, Harlow: Longman.

Mead, L. (1985) *Beyond Entitlement: The Social Obligations of Citizenship*, New York: Free Press.

Means, R. and Langan, M. (1996) 'Charging and quasi-markets in community care: implications for elderly people with dementia', *Social Policy and Administration*, 30(3), pp. 244–262.

Means, R. and Smith, R. (1998) *Community Care: Policy and Practice*, London: Macmillan (2nd edn).

Millar, J. (2001) *The New Deal; The Experience So Far*, York: Joseph Rowntree Foundation.

Monbiot, G. (2000) *Captive State: The Corporate Takeover of Britain*, London: Macmillan.

Morris, J. (1991) *Pride against Prejudice*, London: The Women's Press.

Morris, J. (1993) *Community Care or Independent Living?*, York: Joseph Rowntree Trust.

Morris, J. (1997) 'Care or empowerment? A disability rights perspective', *Social Policy and Administration*, 31(1), pp. 54–60.

Morris, L. (1994) *Dangerous Classes: The underclass and social citizenship*, London: Routledge.

Mulgan, G. (1997) 'Seize the day', *Community Care*, 22–28 May.

Mulhall, S. and Swift, A. (1994) *Liberals and Communitarians*, Oxford: Blackwell.

Murray, C. (1994) *Underclass: The Crisis Deepens*, London: IEA.

NALGO (1989) *Social Work in Crisis*, London: NALGO/University of Southampton.

Neate, P. (2000) *Interview with John Hutton*, available at www.communitycare.co.uk.

NISW (1988) 'Residential Care: A positive choice', *Independent Review of Residential Care* (Wagner Report Part 1), London: HMSO.

Oliver, M. (1996) *Understanding Disability: From Theory to Practice*, London: Macmillan.

Oliver, M. and Barnes, C. (1998) *Disabled People and Social Policy: From Exclusion to Inclusion*, London: Longman,

ONS Omnibus Survey (1997) *Young Carers and their Families*, London: ONS.

Parker, R. A. (1988) 'Children', in L. Sinclair *Residential Care: The Research Reviewed*, London: NISW.

Parker, R. (1995) 'Child care and the personal social services', in Gladstone, D. (ed.) *British Social Welfare*, Cambridge: UCL, pp. 170–182.

Parton, N. (1991) *Governing the Family: Child Care, Child Protection and the State*, London: Macmillan.

Parton, N. (1996a) 'Social theory, social change and social work: an introduction', in Parton, N. (ed.) *Social Theory, Social Change and Social Work*, London: Routledge.

Parton, N. (1996b) 'Social work, risk and the 'blaming system'' in Parton, N (ed.) (1996) *Social Theory, Social Change and Social Work*, London: Routledge.

Parton, N. (ed.) (1996c) *Social Theory, Social Change and Social Work*, London: Routledge.

Parton, N. (ed.) (1997a) *Child Protection: Tensions, Contradictions and Possibilities*, London: Routledge.

Parton, N. (1997b) 'Child protection and family support: current debates and future prospects', in Parton, N. (ed.) *Child Protection and Family Support*, London: Routledge.

Parton, N. and O'Byrne, P. (2000) *Constructive Social Work*, Basingstoke: Macmillan.

Patel, N. (1990) *A 'Race' against Time: Social Service Provision to Black Elders'*, London: Runnymede Trust.

Payne, M. (2000) *Team-work in Multi-professional Care*, London: Macmillan.

Peace, S., Kellaher, L. and Willcocks, D. (1997) *Reevaluating Residential Care*, Buckingham: Open University Press.

Pearson, C. (2000) 'Money talks? Competing discourses in the implementation of direct payments', *Critical Social Policy*, 20(4), pp. 459–479.

Petrie, S. and Wilson, K. (1999) 'Towards the disintegration of child welfare services', *Social Policy and Administration*, 33(2), pp. 181–196.

Phillips, M. (1997) 'Welfare and the common good', in Deacon, A. (ed.) *Stakeholder Welfare*, London: IEA.

Phillipson, C. (1998) *Reconstructing Old Age: New Agendas in Social Theory and Practice*, London: Sage.

Platt, D. (2001) 'Refocusing children's services: evaluation of an initial assessment process', *Child and Family Social Work*, 6, pp. 139-148.

Player, S. and Pollock, A. (2001) 'Long-term care: from public responsibility to private good', *Critical Social Policy*, 21(2), pp. 231–247.

Postle, F. (2000) 'The social work side is disappearing. I guess it started with us being called care managers', *Practice*, 13(2), pp. 13–27.

Powell, F. (2001) *The Politics of Social Work*, London: Sage.

Priestley, M. (1998) 'Discourse and resistance in care assessment: integrated living and community care', *British Journal of Social Work*, 28, pp. 659–673.

Pringle, K. (1998) *Children and Social Welfare in Europe*, Buckingham: Open University Press.

Pritchard, C. (1997) 'Two decades of progress: an international review of child protection services', in Bates, J., Pugh, R. and Thompson, N. *Protecting Children: Challenges and Change*, Aldershot: Arena, pp. 57–75.

Pugh, R. (2000) *Rural Social Work*, Lyme Regis, Dorset: Russell House.

Pugh, R. and Gould, N. (2000) 'Globalization, social work, and social welfare', *European Journal of Social Work*, 3(2), pp. 123–138.

Roberts, T.P (1992) *We Shall Meet on a Beautiful Shore*, Denbigh: Gee and Son.

Rooney, B. (1987) 'Racism and resistance to change: a study of the Black Social Workers Project', Liverpool Social Services Department, Merseyside Area Profile Group, Liverpool.

Royal Commission on Long Term Care (1999) *With Respect to Old Age,* Cm. 4192, London: HMSO.

Sapey, B. (1995) 'Disabling homes: a study of the housing needs of disabled people in Cornwall', *Disability and Society*, 10(1), pp. 71–86.

Save The Children Fund (1995) *You're on Your Own*, London: Save The Children Fund.

Schwehr, B. (2001) 'Human rights and social services', in Cull, L. and Roche, J. *The Law and Social Work: Contemporary Issues for Practice,* London: Palgrave.

Seebohm Report (1968) *Report of the Committee on Local Authority and Allied Personal Social Services*, Cmnd 3703, London: HMSO.

Servian, R. (1996) *Theorising Empowerment: Individual Power and Community Care,* Bristol: Policy Press.

Shaw, I. (2000) 'Mental health', in Hill, M. (ed.) *Local Authority Social Services: An Introduction*, Oxford: Blackwell.

Simm, M. (1995) 'Aiming high', *Community Care*, 2–8 November, pp. 16–20.

Sinclair, I. (1988) 'Residential care for elderly people', in NISW, *Residential Care: a Positive Choice, Independent Review of Residential Care* (Wagner Report Part 1), London: HMSO.

Sinclair, I. and Gibbs, I. (1998) *Children's Homes: A Study in Diversity*, Chichester: Wiley.

Smith, C. (2001) 'Trust and confidence: possibilities for social work in "high modernity"', *British Journal of Social Work*, 31(2), pp. 287–305.

Smith, R., Gaster, L., Harrison, L., Martin, L., Means, R. and Thistlethwaite, P. (1993) *Working Together for Better Community Care*, Bristol: SAUS Study No. 7.

Social Exclusion Unit (2000) *Preventing Social Exclusion,* London: Cabinet Office

Social Services Committee (1985) *Community Care with Special Reference to Adult Mentally Ill and Mentally Handicapped People*, HC 13–1, London: HMSO.

Social Services Inspectorate (1997) *When Leaving Home is also Leaving Care*, London: Department of Health.

Social Services Inspectorate/Audit Commission (1998*) Getting the Best from Social Services: Learning the Lessons from the Joint Reviews*, Abingdon: Audit Commission.

Social Services Inspectorate/Audit Commission (2000*) People need People,* Abingdon, Audit Commission.

Stanley, N. (1999) 'User–practitioner transactions in the new culture of community care', *British Journal of Social Work*, 29, pp. 417–435.

Stein, M. and Carey, K. (1986) *Leaving Care*, Oxford: Blackwell.

Stevenson, O. and Parsloe, P. (1993) *Community Care and Empowerment*, York: Joseph Rowntree Trust.

Sullivan, M. (1996) *The Development of the British Welfare State*, Hemel Hempstead: Prentice Hall/Harvester Wheatsheaf.

Taylor-Gooby, P. (1996) 'The United Kingdom: radical departures and political consensus', in George, V. and Taylor-Gooby, P. (eds) *European Welfare Policy: Squaring the Welfare Circle*, London: Macmillan.

Thane, P. (1996) *Foundations of the Welfare State*, London: Longman (2nd edn).

Thompson, N. (1998) *Promoting Equality: Challenging Discrimination and Oppression in the Human Services*, London: Macmillan.

Townsend, P. (1964) *The Last Refuge*, London: Routledge & Kegan Paul.

Toynbee, P. and Walker, D. (2001) *Did Things get Better? An Audit of Labour's Successes and Failures*, London: Penguin.

Tunstill, J. (1997) 'Implementing the family support clauses of the 1989 Children Act: legislative, professional and organisational obstacles', in Parton, N. (ed.) *Child Protection and Family Support: Tensions, Contradictions and Possibilities*, London: Routledge.

Twigg, J. (2000) *Bathing: The Body and Community Care*, London: Routledge.

Ungerson, C. (1997) 'Give them money: is cash a route to empowerment', *Social Policy and Administration*, 31(1). pp. 45–53.

Utting, W. (1997) *People Like Us*, London: HMSO.

Walker, A. (1989) 'Community care', in M. McCarthy (ed.) *The New Politics of Welfare*, London: Macmillan.

Walker, A. (1993) 'Community care policy: from consensus to conflict', in Bornat, J., Johnson, J., Periera, C. and Pilgrim, D. (1993) *Community Care: A Reader*, 2nd edn, London: Palgrave.

Waqar, A. and Atkins, C. (1996) *Race and Community Care*, Buckingham: Open University Press.

Watson, L. and Harker, M. (1993) *Community Care Planning: A Model for Housing Need Assessment*, London: National Federation of Housing Associations/Institute of Housing.

Webb, A. and Wistow, G. (1987) *Social Work, Social Care and Social Planning: The Personal Social Services Since Seebohm*, London: Longman.

Wheal, C. (2001) 'Going concerns', *Guardian*, 2 May.

Williams, F. (1989) *Social Policy: A Critical Introduction*, Cambridge: Polity Press.

Williams, F. (1998) 'Agency and structure revisited: rethinking poverty and social exclusion' in Barry, M. and Hallett, C. *Social Exclusion and Social Work: Issues in Theory and Practice*, Lyme Regis, Dorset: Russell House.

Williams Report (1967) *Caring for People: Staffing Residential Homes*, London: Allen and Unwin.

Wilson, A. and Beresford, P. (2000) '"Anti-oppressive practice": emancipation or appropriation?', *British Journal of Social Work*, 30, pp. 553–573.

Wilson, G. (2000) *Understanding Old Age: Critical and Global Perspectives*, London: Sage.

Wistow, G., Knapp, M., Hardy, B., Forder, J., Kendall, J. and Manning, R. (1996) *Social Care Markets*, Buckingham: Open University Press.

Index